How and why we get Alzheimer's disease

Norbert Wrobel, who lives in Berlin, studied medicine and was licensed as a doctor in 1984. In a broad-based basic university education at the Freie Universität (FU) Berlin, he subsequently specialized in internal medicine, intensive care medicine, emergency medicine and later also in geriatric medicine. Since then he has worked in in-patient hospital treatment. His current research focus is on chronic degenerative diseases of the brain, heart and skeletal muscles.

With regard to the sporadic form of Alzheimer's disease, a reduction to molecular-biological or genetic processes does not sufficiently contribute to the understanding of its development. Its pathogenesis only becomes clearer from an emergent perspective, a critical examination of the existing hypotheses on the development of the disease and the inclusion of fundamental scientific findings. Against an extremely complex background, the energetic factor stands out. The efficiency of some processes in cellular energy use and production points to principles of quantum information. In this context, potentially new diagnostic and therapeutic methods are discussed.

Correspondence address:

science@norbertwrobel.de

Note:

The numbers in brackets in the text refer to an entry in the bibliography.

Norbert Wrobel

How and why we get Alzheimer's disease

Complexity dynamics of a chronic disease triggered by mitochondrial energetic dysfunction

Approaching quantum information theory in biologic matter

Published 2023 by
Klaus-Dieter Sedlacek

Scientific Library Vol. 22

Bibliographic Information of Die Deutsche Bibliothek: Die Deutsche Bibliothek lists this publication in the German National Bibliography; detailed bibliographic data are available on the Internet at http://dnb.ddb.de.

Editor: Klaus-Dieter Sedlacek
Cover design, book typesetting: Sedlacek
Internet: https://klaus-sedlacek.de

© 2023 Norbert Wrobel
Herstellung und Verlag: BoD - Books on Demand, Norderstedt.
ISBN: 978-3-7578-0382-7

Tabel of contents

1 A different view on the origin of the sporadic form of Alzheimer's disease: Neuronal mitochondrial energetics

1.1 Introduction

There are various entities attributed to Alzheimer's disease. A purely familial form of the disease differs from the sporadically occurring one. The latter appears mainly in old age and has a multifactorial genesis.

Accordingly, the sporadic form of Alzheimer's disease is an age-related neurodegenerative disorder of the brain. Clinically, it is characterized by a progressive loss of cognitive abilities and associated behavioral and neuropsychological symptoms. Consistent with the amyloid theory, its pathognomy results from protein misfolding of extracellularly stored amyloid (Aß) plaques and intracellular neurofibrils formed by hyperphosphorylated tau protein. This cascade is partly hypothetical (1) and therefore controversial. In particular, the circumstances of the mechanisms that lead to the degradation of a neuron have not yet been fully elucidated. Also why the presence of plaques and the onset of cognitive impairment are not necessarily correlated. Above all, cognitive abilities cannot be significantly improved after therapeutic administration of biologics for plaques reduction or removal, which is tantamount to a falsification of the corresponding hypothesis.

This is in contrast to the hypothesis of nerve cell damage due to mitochondrial bioenergetic dysfunction (2). In terms of development history, the dynamic aspect is to be emphasized. The effects of mutations in the mitochondrial DNA, aging and, in particular, the energy supply of a cell are taken into account. Mitochondria are considered the power plants of a cell and cover the high energy requirements of neurons in the brain.

In the case of multifactorial upregulated oxidative phosphorylation, the rate of reactive oxygen species increases the likelihood of mutations in mitochondrial DNA. The resulting aging of a cell and the change in the specific energy-supplying property of the mitochondria have a degeneratively destructive effect on the neurons of the brain. They become senescent or die from programmed cell death.

All life derives from complex processes and requires only a few ingredients to form robustly. According to recent findings, animal and plant life originally arose through quantum mechanical effects such as "tunneling" or "coherence", while competition and stress were constant drivers of natural selection. A milestone in this development was the emergence of the eukaryotes and thus the mitochondria. Over time, the latter became the key energy supplier of a cell and were also able to process, store and use information. Whether dysfunctional mitochondria may be at the forefront of the cascade in the sporadic form of Alzheimer's disease is the subject of this systematic review. Nevertheless, the result could indicate a typical chicken-and-egg problem. Then the question of the actual substance immediately arises.

1.2 What is currently known about Alzheimer's disease?

1.2.1 Amyloid cascade

Alzheimer's disease regularly presents as a predominantly age-related, progressive and neurodegenerative disorder. As the disease stride ahead orientation, communication skills, autobiographical identity and personality traits become impaired. Histologically, Amyloid-β(Aß)-plaques are found extracellularly in nerve tissue.

They consist of misfolded ß-amyloid peptide. In contrast, neurofibrils of hyperphosphorylated tau proteins are localized intracellularly.

Amyloid is a protein-polysaccharide complex of diverse origin. To date, more than 25 such proteins of different structure and function have been described, including immunoglobulins, serum transport proteins, apolipoproteins, hormones and proteases. Normally, amyloid is present in dissolved form in blood serum. A pathological situation results from an overproduction of misfolded and dysfunctional amyloidogenic proteins. Due to a conformational change of the original protein with conversion from α-helical structures to β-sheet structures, gives rise to insoluble complexes in form of microscopic fibers. These can no longer be adequately degraded or excreted and are therefore deposited in interstitial or even functional tissues (3).

In Alzheimer's disease, hard amyloid plaques are found extracellularly in the brain. ß-Amyloid (Aß) is a protein fragment of the amyloid precursor protein (APP) that is also involved in the formation of junctions between neurons. APP can be cleaved by three different enzymes: physiologically by an α-secretase close to the membrane, under which its n-terminal end enters the extracellular space as soluble sAPP and is normally disposed of. In contrast, there is an amyloidogenic pathway via β-secretase, which, as a membrane-bound enzyme, cuts off APP in the extracellular space and releases an extracellular, soluble fragment. Then the transmembrane region of APP is separated out by γ-secretase. Faulty cleavage at the n-terminal and c-terminal end by β-secretase and γ-secretase gives rise in β-amyloids: amyloid Aβ-1-40 and Aβ-1-43 as well as the neurotoxic Aβ-1-42.

These counteract all other defense mechanisms and therefore remain in place. Extracellularly, $A\beta$-1-42 molecules initially form smaller, oligomeric aggregates. They then polymerize into large, hard and insoluble amyloid plaques between neurons, which eventually become surrounded by abnormal neuronal processes and glia cells. Immune cells originating from microglia are activated and then trigger inflammatory tissue-damaging reactions in the brain. Similarly, amyloid is deposited in the walls of small blood vessels. Inflammatory processes reduce their permeability with negative effects on the oxygen and energy supply (4). According to recent findings, β-amyloid also accumulates in neurons. The relevance of this finding has not been conclusively clarified. These may be relics of the immune system active in the brain (5).

In addition, $A\beta$-1-42 plaques cause increased permeability of $Ca2^+$ ions in neuronal membranes affecting synaptic signaling, as shown in the hippocampus. This impairs short and long-term memory. Otherwise, $Ca2^+$ ions are essential for intracellular signaling cascades. Increased influx can activate kinases, e.g., microtubules affinity-regulating kinase (MARK), which then hyperphosphorylate tau protein, a microtubule associated protein (MAP). This process gradually leads to their detachment from the cytoskeletal structure, resulting in aggregation into neurofibrillary tangles. The tau protein is responsible for maintaining the structure of the microtubules. Microtubules form the cytoskeleton by transporting cell nutrients and other molecules throughout the cell. Excessive loading of tau protein with phosphate groups disrupts many stabilization and transport processes until finally the cytoskeleton with the microtubular structures collapses and causes neuronal cell death (6).

Taken together, these processes lead to the destruction of tissue architecture. The brain shrinks by up to 20% of its original volume, while the vertebral sulci on its surface deepen and the cerebral ventricles expand. Morphologically it atrophies. Gaps left by the death of neurons are filled by proliferating glial supporting tissue. Topographically, the hippocampal region is affected early. Cortical areas of the temporal and frontal lobes are involved in processing. Later also deeper brain structures, accompanied by the destruction of synapses, which are used for the transmission and processing of information. In the lower cerebral cortex is the basal nucleus Meynert, whose nerve cells produce the messenger substance acetylcholine. If cells in this nucleus die, acetylcholine loses its function as a neurotransmitter. Finally, full-fledged neurodegenerative Alzheimer's disease is characterized by severe brain and mental disorders. These include, among others:

- memory
- recall
- language
- faculty of thought and ability to judge
- recognition
- object handling
- orientation.

In the course of the disease, the nature of the human being also changes. Distrust, aggression, restlessness, anxiety, depression, delusions, disinhibition, affect lability or apathy and loss of interest occur across a broad intra- and inter-individual spectrum (7) (8).

1.2.2 Diagnostic possibilities

Adequate biomarkers are suitable for preclinically indicating pathological changes in the brain. From a molecular-biological point of view, a ratio of amyloid-Aβ-1-42 peptides and tau protein from cerebrospinal fluid in the context of imaging techniques such as magnetic resonance imaging (MRI), fluorodeoxyglucose (FDG), positron emission tomography (PET) or the new methods of in-vivo amyloid PET imaging are considered relevant biomarkers in Alzheimer's disease. These are complemented by the immune receptor sTrem2 as an expression of increased activity of the microglia (9). In addition, there are biometric methods for monitoring the progression of neuropsychological disorders.

1.2.3 Therapeutic options

Alzheimer's patients currently have four synthetically produced active ingredients available: the three acetylcholinesterase inhibitors donepezil, rivastigmine and galantamine and the NMDA antagonist memantine. They may delay the decline in mental capacity, alleviate some of the symptoms and slightly improve everyday life skills. Non-drug therapies encompass a range of therapeutic and individualized treatment options. Molecular biological and genetic or epigenetic therapeutic strategies aim, among other things, at the use of antibodies or active and passive immunization or signaling in the immune system (10). A breakthrough has not yet been achieved (11).

1.2.4 Mitochondrial aspects

Impaired function affects the mitochondria's ability to provide sufficient energy in the form of ATP for essential life processes.

This is mainly due to mutations in mitochondrial DNA (mtDNA), which are stored separately in several thousand copies in mitochondria in cells with high energy expenditure such as neurons. Indications of mitochondrial dysfunction in the patho-genesis of Alzheimer's disease are reduced activity of the three rel-evant enzyme complexes of the citric acid cycle, pyruvate dehyd-rogenase, isocitrate dehydrogenase and α-ketoglutarate dehydro-genase (12) as well as a reduced activity of complexes I, III and IV (13). Additional 20 point mutations in the genes of the mtDNA-encoded cytochrome coxidase subunits I, II and III have been identified in Alzheimer's patients (14).

In addition, functions are influenced by direct interactions, e.g., via APP. Mitochondria are made up of around 1.500 different proteins, most of which have to migrate before they become ef-fective. This import takes place with the help of so-called signal se-quences as small protein attachments. Normally, these are re-moved again after entry, but this can be hindered by deposited amyloid beta protein fragments. This leads to an accumulation of unfinished proteins that are unstable and can only fulfill their function in energy metabolism to a limited extent (15).

Ultimately, symptoms and disease-related consequences arise from a complex energetic dysfunction (2) similar to those ob-served in chronic neurodegenerative diseases. For example, the gene expression profile is the pattern of gene activity at the level at which mtDNA mutations induce brain dysfunction, similar to the profiles found in Alzheimer's, Parkinson's or Huntington's disease. All of these findings suggest an association between disease devel-opment and energy-deficient mitochondrial dysfunction (16).

1.2.4.1 Side view: Quality control in protein folding

Protein folding is a complex and error-prone process that requires quality control. All secretory proteins synthesized in a cell are systematically directed to the endoplasmic re-ticulum (ER). The quality assurance of the proteins is car-

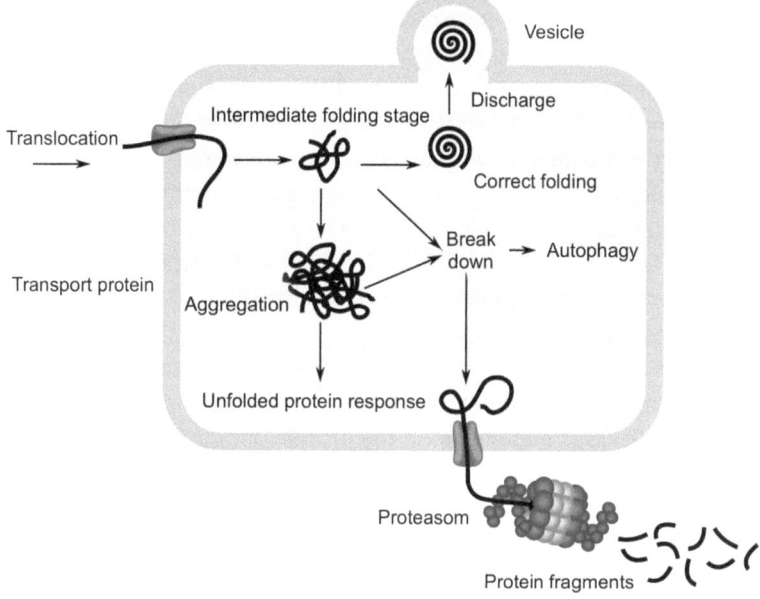

Fig. 1: Scheme of protein quality control in the endoplasmic reticulum.
CCO Armin Kübelbeck.

ried out using a multi-stage system in three phases: In the first phase the proteins are checked by proofreading. In the second phase attempts are made to fold still unfolded (Fig. 1) proteins with the help of chaperones (17). These accelerate correct folding without becoming part of the protein structure themselves. In the subsequent third phase of quality assurance, chaperones help to identify faulty proteins. If the folded protein is recognized as correct, it is removed from the ER by vesicle and transported to its destination. Chaperones also serve as platforms for the assignment of proteins to specific cellular compartments and for assembling individual protein components into higher-order structures (10).

Misfolded proteins are funneled into the cytoplasm as a transport protein and broken down into fragments in a proteasome. The proteasome is a protein found in the cytoplasm and in nucleus of eukaryotes.

Amorphous aggregates are disassembled into cellular components and recycled through autophagy. Accumulation of misfolded proteins in the endoplasmic reticulum induces a cellular stress response associated with translational suppression and increased chaperones synthesis.

Statistically, 30% of folded proteins are defective and even more in complex cases. This scrap typically disintegrates into fragments in about ten minutes (18). If degradation fails or if it is misjudged by protein quality control, the result is defective protein synthesis, which can cause various diseases depending on the protein. Either toxic deposits form or, in the worst case, insoluble aggregates or there is a loss of function due to the lack of functional proteins in the cell or at the target site in the organism. For example, amyloid is an insoluble deposit in the form of small fibers (β-fibrils) (19).

1.3 Characteristics of cellular mitochondria

The evolution of life from prebiotic molecules to a living cell probably occurred via self-replicating RNA through enzymatic activity of proteins and through DNA acting as the genetic code. The early bacteria and archaea finally emerged from LUCA (=Last universal common ancestor) (Fig. 2).

According to the endosymbiont theory (20), the first eucytes are the result of the fusion of methanogenic archaea with α-proteobacteria (α-PB) capable of oxidative phosphorylation: by not digesting α-PB after phagocytosis, a symbiotic relationship developed that enabled the eucyte as a host cell to better adapt to different environmental conditions. During evolution into modern eukaryotes, their genome was fused to that of α-PB by partial lateral gene transfer. In the process, α-proteobacteria lost their

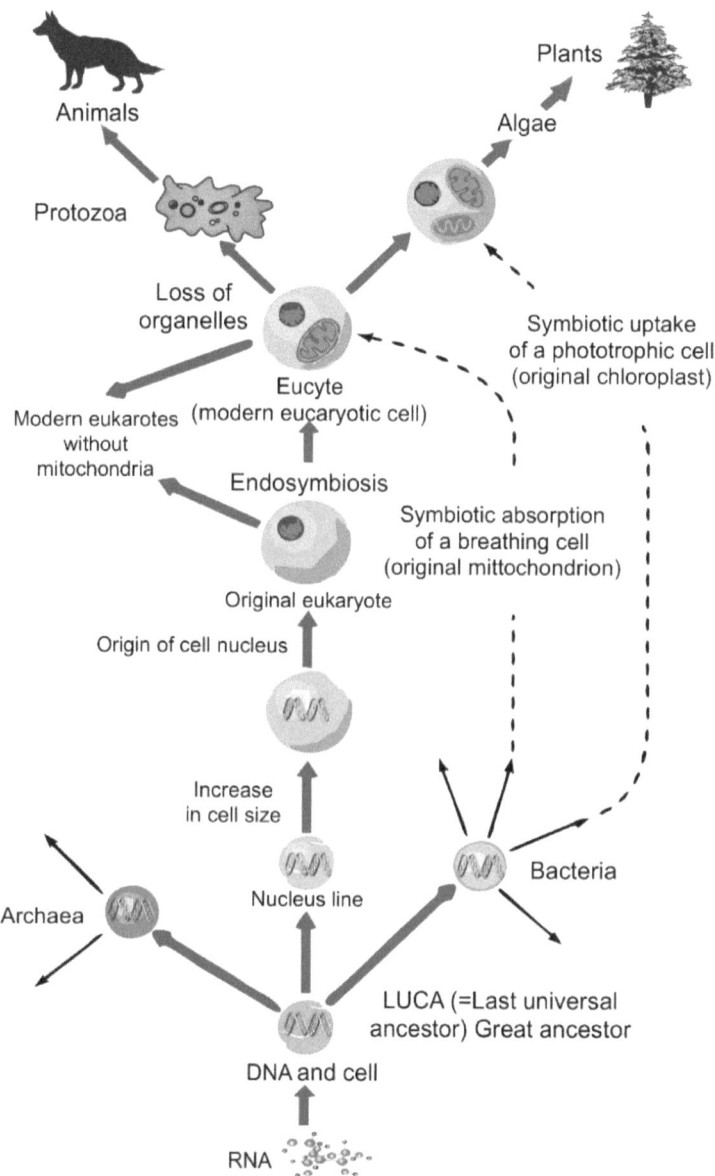

Fig. 2: Last universal common ancestor (Luca).
Grafic Sedlacek

structural integrity and evolved into an organelle with new functionality to become the power plant of a cell. As a relic of the fusion process, a mitochondrion, unlike other organelles, has a double membrane and its own extrachromosomal DNA (mtDNA). In contrast, the chromosomal nuclear DNA (nDNA) of eukaryotes contains parts from the genome of archaea and α-proteobacteria.

Human mtDNA contains 37 genes (nDNA over 20.000) and forms a closed, circular and double-stranded DNA macromolecule of almost 17.000 base pairs (nDNA 3.3 billion). It contains 2 ribosomal rRNA, 22 transfer tRNA responsible for transcription, translation and replication and 13 protein complexes that collectively code for energy production in the respiratory chain. A lively exchange of information takes place between the nuclear and mitochondrial DNA. Most mitochondrial proteins are encoded by nuclear nDNA, synthesized in the cytoplasm by mRNA and then imported into the mitochondria. Although mtDNA contains far fewer genes compared to nDNA, it plays a key role in a complex network of vital biochemical processes.

It is understandable that mitochondria no longer replicate themselves. Their intracellular propagation occurs by budding as local growth of a daughter organelle. During cell division, existing mitochondria are distributed to daughter cells. Most of the proteins required for mitochondria regeneration are synthesized in the cytosol, quality controlled by chaperones and then transported into the mitochondria. How often the mitochondria of a eukaryotic cell propagate depends on its energy requirements. Cells with high energy expenditure, such as skeletal muscle or nerve cells, have several thousand mitochondria or fused systems. Demand is met through coordinated fission and fusion processes (21). Another peculiarity is that a mitochondrion itself can have multiple copies of circular mtDNA - and a single cell several thousand of them.

1.4 Energy production: Respiratory chain

Some cells obtain their energy from the metabolism of carbohydrates, fat or proteins. The necessary enzymes act in the cytoplasm of prokaryotes and in the inner mitochondrial membrane of eukaryotes (Fig. 3).

For example, the degradation of glucose to carbon dioxide and water using oxygen, yielding energy in the form of ATP

$$C_6 H_{12} O_6 + 6 O_2 \rightarrow 6 CO_2 + 6 H_2 O + xATP$$

is accomplished by oxidative phosphorylation (OxPhos) as the final step in traversing the respiratory chain. OxPhos accompanies the cytoplasmic glycolysis up to the citrate acid cycle located in the matrix. The resulting acceptors NADH and FADH donate electrons for oxidative phosphorylation reactions.

All thirteen mtDNA-encoded proteins are part of the mitochondrial enzyme complexes responsible for oxidative phosphorylation. Its site of action is the inner mitochondrial membrane. The specific function of the respiratory chain is performed by nuclear-encoded proteins imported from the nucleus. The latter also take on other metabolic tasks and regulate expression of mitochondrial proteins.

Glucose is utilized by oxidizing hydrogen to water in a fractionated exergonic oxyhydrogen reaction

$$O_2 + 4H^+ + 4e^- = 2 H_2 O$$

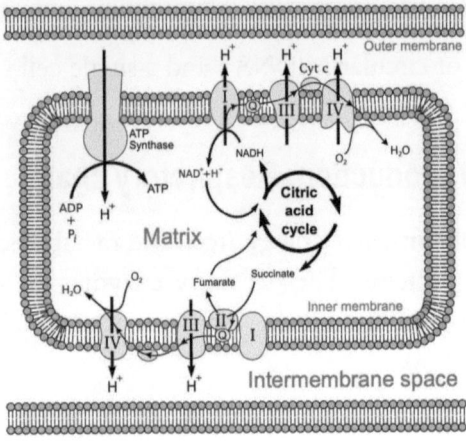

Fig. 3: Schematic representation of the respiratory chain with complexes (I, II, III and IV)
And ATP synthase (complex V) in the inner membrane of mitochondria.Mitochondrial electron
transport chain.
Klaus Hoffmeier, public domain

thereby releasing carbon dioxide. This is achieved through a cascaded transfer of electrons across a series of redox systems organized into integral membrane complexes (complex I-IV). Complexes I, III and IV use the energy to pump protons from the mitochondrial matrix into the intermembrane space. The resulting electrochemical proton gradient generates a proton motor force. The ATP synthase located in complex V uses this power through oxidative phosphorylation to synthesize adenosine triphosphate (ATP) from adenosine diphosphate (ADP) and phosphate (=chemiosmotic synthesis). The hydrogen and electron carriers Ubiquinone (Coenzyme Q) and Cytochrome C stored in the inner mitochondrial membrane, are involved in this cascade process.

1.4.1.1 Side view: Electron transport chain (ETC)

An electron transport chain, as illustrated in the respiratory chain, represents a biological process of electron-transferring molecules with energy transfer from donors to acceptors. This process is characterized by its highly efficient energy yield. Photosynthesis, discussed in

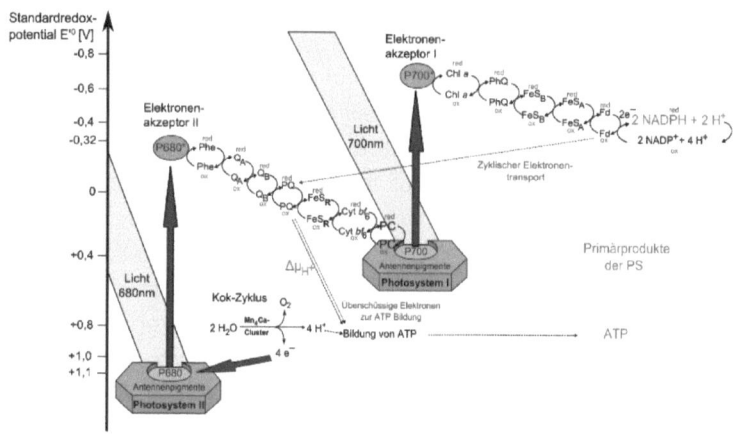

Fig. 4: The Z-scheme of the light reaction in oxygenic photosynthesis.
Lanzi, public domain

more detail below, has been well studied in this regard (Fig. 4).

Glucose and oxygen are formed during photosynthesis from water and carbon dioxide under the influence of massless photons emitted by the sun (=electromagnetic wave, energy):

$$6\ H_2O + 6\ CO_2 + \text{light quanta} \rightarrow 6\ O_2 + C_6H_{12}O_6$$

Phototrophic organisms use antenna complexes. Light quanta are absorbed by special antenna pigments of the photosystem I in the thylakoid membrane of the chloroplast. The energy thus gained is passed on to the photosynthetic pigments such as carotenoids or chlorophylls a, b or c, which are arranged around a reaction center, the light-collecting complex and collected from them. Photosynthetic activity can be detected in different ranges of visible light that correspond to the absorption maxima of the photosynthetic pigments.

All antenna pigments have a system that allows electrons to transition from a ground state to an excited state by absorbing energy. The arrangement of the pigments allows the excited state to be transferred to a neighboring photosynthetic pigment of the light-harvesting complex. This process continues until the excitation energy reaches the reaction center with the absorption maximum corresponding to the longest wave length, belonging to chlorophyll a. The electron transport chain then set in motion releases an excited electron, which is captured by an acceptor. For example, electrons can be transferred to $NADH^+$ via ferredoxin and, together with the protons from the photolysis of water, cause the formation of $NADH+H^+$. The acceptor $NADH^+$ is reduced by absorbing the hydrogen ions from the photolysis. ATP is then obtained according to the principle of chemiosmotic coupling.

The energy now stored in ATP is used by the enzyme ribulose-1,5-bisphosphate-carboxylase/-oxygenase (RuBisCO) to form glucose or starch. Only RuBisCo is able to absorb carbon dioxide. It initiates carbon dioxide fixation in the Calvin cycle, after which the dark reaction of photosynthesis is set in motion. RuBisCO itself only acts enzymatically when stimulated by a light-dependent activase.

1.4.1.2 Side view: Special features of porphyrins and enzymes

Porphyrins

Porphyrins are organic chemical pigments and are found in almost all organisms. They are important in many metabolic processes, are involved in various transport actions, for example for oxygen or electrons or develop catalytic activity as coenzymes. Legitimate analogies between plant and animal eukaryotes result from their evolutionarily history (Fig. 5).

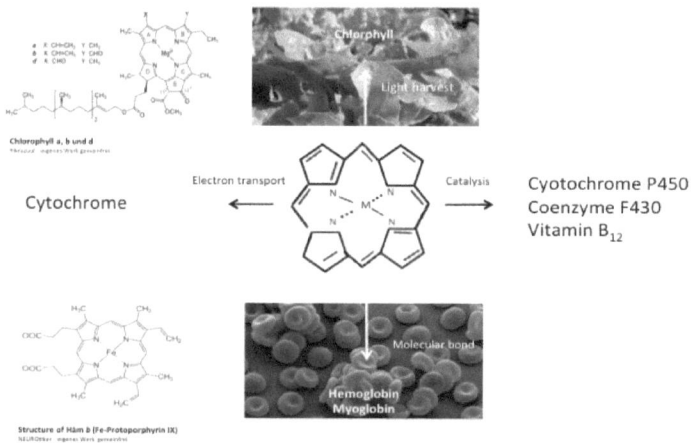

Fig. 5: Various functions of metalloporphyrins in nature.
Graphic Wrobel

Porphyrins tend to form chelates with metal ions. In hemoglobin the central metal ion is divalent iron ($Fe2^+$), in chlorophyll it is divalent magnesium ($Mg2^+$), resulting in different colors. The leaf green comes from chlorophyll. When withering, the hue changes to yellow. However, the special foliage coloration in autumn is due to carotenoids. Blood, on the other hand, is normally red and can be traced back to the hemin of hemoglobin, the blood pigment. A bruise occurs when red blood initially leaks from the capillaries into the connective tissue and coagulates there. Over time, the colors change from green to yellow until the once blue spot has finally disappeared.

The main function of hemoglobin is to take up O_2 from the inhaled air in the lungs and pass it to the tissues and organs of a body. The release of CO_2 via the exhaled air from the lungs is directly related to this. The process of absorbing or releasing O_2 or CO_2 takes place loosely at the

23

iron-metal complex of the porphyrin. Intracellularly, O_2 is required in the respiratory chain for the fractionated oxy-hydrogen reaction to generate ATP energy. The CO_2 produced during degradation of glucose is coupled to the hemin and is smoked off with the exhaled air.

Porphyrins also transfer electrons from one region to another. This process can be followed particularly clearly during "light harvest" in the light-harvesting complex (see photosynthesis). An expression of the high efficiency is a practically heat-loss-free transmission of the light energy of the sun for the chemiosmotic production of ATP.

Enzymes

Enzymes are biocatalysts. Without them, most biochemical reactions in organisms would occur at negligible speeds. The activation energy is relevant as an energetic barrier that must be overcome by the reactants in a chemical reaction. As a special ability, enzymes reduce the activation energy and thereby accelerate the conversion of substances. The substrate as the starting material is bound in the active center of the enzyme in an energetically unfavorable transition state that is stabilized by interactions. With this enzyme-substrate-complex, substrates are rapidly converted into reaction products. After their release from the complex, the enzyme returns to its initial state. Enzymes are characterized by a high substrate and reaction specificity. They select suitable substrates from numerous substances and catalyze exactly one of many conceivable reactions.

The catalytically active center forms the structural basis for catalysis and specificity. At this point, enzymes bind to the substrate and thus enter an activated mode.

The special spatial structure of the active center only allows the binding of a structurally exactly matching substrate (lock-and-key principle). There is also another less rigid model (induced fit model), where the active site can

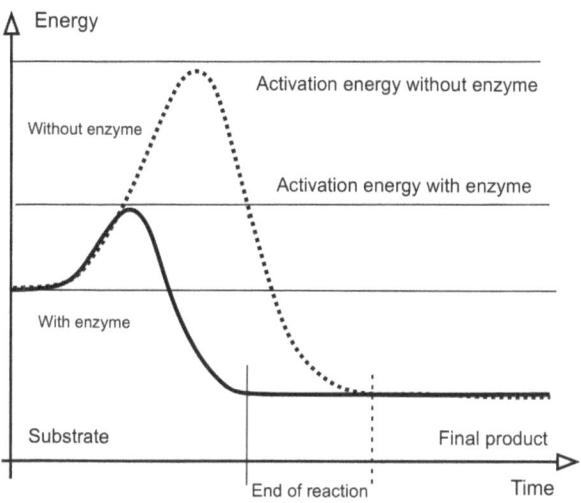

Fig. 6: Energy-time diagram of an enzymatic reaction: The required activation energy is reduced compared to the uncatalyzed reaction. Reactions with enzymes accelerate the biochemical process (not to
scale).
Grafic Sedlacek

be suitably shaped by interaction with the substrate. This
flexibility is advantageous if, for example, a substance on
the substrate is no longer recognized due to small differ-
ences in the enzyme's spatial structure or charge distribution. For example, glucokinase accepts glucose as a substrate, but its stereoisomer galactose does not. On the
other hand, alcohol dehydrogenase with extended substrate specificity degrades other alcohols besides ethanol.
Hexokinase IV also accepts hexoses other than glucose as
a substrate.

1.5   Mutation: Effect on mitochondrial DNA

The complex structure, inefficient DNA repair system, frequent
cycles of replication and high flux of oxygen radicals along the
neighboring respiratory chain make mtDNA susceptible to muta-

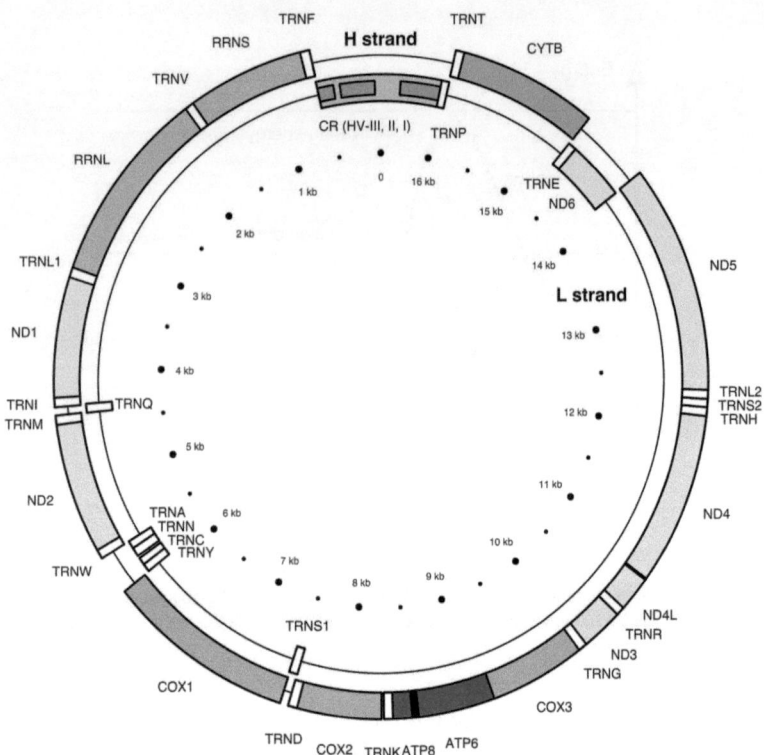

Fig. 7: Map of the human mitochondrial DNA genome. The 16,569 bp long human mitochondrial genome with the protein-coding, ribosomal RNA and transfer RNA genes.
By Emmanuel Douzery. Own work, CC BY-SA 4.0, https://commons.wikimedia.org/w/index.php?curid=46726514

tions at a rate 10 to 20 times higher than assumed in the nuclear genome (22).

Changes due to the accumulation of mtDNA-associated mutations affect the post-mitotic tissue. The mitochondrial genomes of all mtDNA mutations are recorded in the MITOMAP database (23), which allows the assignment of very different patterns of disorders. From this, a tissue-specific manifestation of diseases can be derived, which results in particular from the energetic roles and specific tasks of different tissues or organs. These primarily include skeletal muscles, heart and brain, but also kidneys or, for example, the visual process of the eyes (24).

1.5.1.1 Side view: Mutation, Methylation

Mutation changes the genetic material, detectable in genes, chromosomes and genomes. The probability of a mutation occurring is significantly increased by mutagens, including chemical substances, radioactivity, UV-radiation or X-rays. From evolutionary point of view, on the other hand, mutation occurs randomly and undirectedly, with beneficial or detrimental or unchanged effects on an individual.

Along with adenine, guanine and thymine, cytosine is one of the four nucleic bases of DNA. They form two coiled strands and are connected by hydrogen bonds. A hydrogen atom consists of a single positively charged atomic nucleus, usually containing one proton, no neutrons and a negatively charged electron e^-.

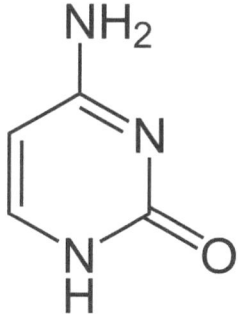

Fig. 8: Structural formula of cytosine

The -NH2 group of cytosine is a common amino group in biological compounds and belongs to the bases. Normally, the binding energy of hydrogen and nitrogen in the amino group is so large that no ions can be released from this compound. However, if, exceptionally, a release occurs, the amino group (-NH2) splits off. However, the release of an H^+ ion and the formation of a new compound is only possible over extremely short distances. In the case of cytosine, this is achieved by the neighboring N atom forming an NH bond together with the emitted H^+ ion. The original double bond to the N atom is broken. The amino group NH^-, decimated by one hydrogen atom, finds water molecules H_2O in the immediate vicinity as reaction partners:

$$NH^- + H_2O \rightarrow O^- + NH_3$$

The resulting NH_3 group has no vacancies in its electron-orbitals. It no longer binds to the cytosine and goes into solution as ammonia, while O^- forms a double bond with the pyrimidine backbone. The result of this reaction is uracil:

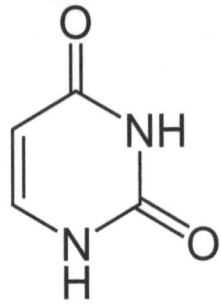

Fig. 9 Structural formula of uracil

Uracil is normally found only in RNA, while its counterpart in DNA is thymine. Uracil in DNA alters the genetic code and becomes a mutation in this form if not recognized by the cell's repair mechanisms.

Like individual genes, large chromosomal regions or entire chromosomes can also show different DNA methylation structure patterns. The resulting altered gene expression without altered DNA sequences is summarized under the term epigenetics. In contrast to the statistical information of DNA, epigenetics stands for dynamic types of information in the interaction of cell components and environmental factors or as an expression of hereditary genesis.

DNA methylation activated by DNA-methyltransferase modifies DNA without causing mutations. For example, the transcription rate altered or the development from zygote to embryo can be influenced. Genes that are no longer required at later stages of development or for certain cell types are methylated and thus silenced, which means that transcription comes to a standstill (25). Conversely, genes that have been silenced are switched on again by demethylation. Dysregulations that occur in the interaction of the promoters of onco genes or tumor suppressor genes are suspected to be causative for cancerogenesis.

1.6 Damage: Oxidative stress, reactive oxygen species, aging

Free radical theory states that oxidative stress leads to aging: the high flux of oxygen radicals along the neighboring respiratory chain makes mtDNA susceptible to mutations at rates up to 20 times higher than assumed in the nuclear genome (22). The mtDNA mutations recorded in the MITOMAP database (23) can be used to assign patterns of disturbances resulting from the energetic roles or specific tasks of tissues or organs. When bioenergetic dysfunction develops, it is associated with both normal aging and chronic degenerative diseases. The brain, heart and skeletal muscles are in particular affected (24).

1.6.1 Reactive oxygen species

Reactive oxygen species (ROS) are formed by normal cellular reactions in aerobic organisms (Fig. 10). In addition to singlet oxygen, ROS contain intermediates formed when oxygen is reduced to water: superoxide anion radicals (O_2), hydrogen peroxide (H_2O_2) and hydroxyl radicals (OH). Hypochloride (HOCl), peroxyl radicals (ROO), alkoxyl radicals (RO) and nitric oxide (NO) are also commonly present. Oxidation and destruction processes by these ROS affect all biological macromolecules, such as lipids, especially those in cell membranes, proteins and DNA, leading to irreversible cell damage.

Hydroxyl radicals are of particular importance for cytotoxic effects because they are the only ROS that can react directly with biological macromolecules.

Oxidative stress and ROS are ubiquitous in biological systems. Normally, ROS are not formed enzymatically by chemical, photo-

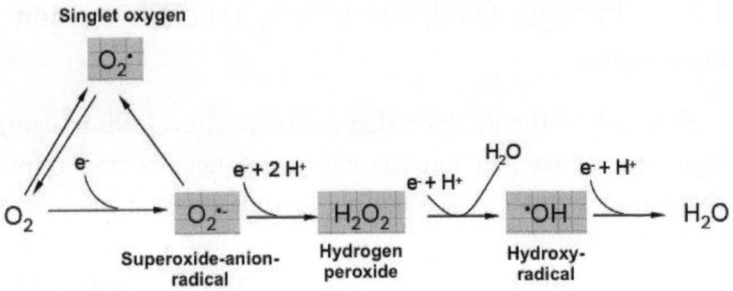

Fig. 10: The activated forms of oxygen. Shown are the forms which are formed by the addition of protons after the absorption of an electron.

chemical and electron transfer reactions or as by-products of endogenous enzymatic reactions, phagocytosis and inflammation. Imbalances in ROS homeostasis caused by antioxidant enzymes or non-enzymatic antioxidant networks, increase oxidative stress and affect biomacromolecules such as lipids, proteins or DNA. While some ROS are important for intracellular signaling and oxidative metabolism is mainly beneficial for normal cell function, elevated ROS levels have been implicated in stress-sensitive signaling, toxicity, oncogenesis, but also neurodegeneration (26). Combined with age- and disease-related loss of mitochondrial function, altered metal homeostasis and reduced antioxidant defenses, synaptic activity and neurotransmission are directly affected, contributing to cognitive dysfunction (27).

1.6.2   Aging

Various theories have been formulated that point to molecular mechanisms or evolutionary processes as the basis of aging:

- ▤   replicative senescence as a cellular aging model (Hayflick limit)

- apoptosis and cellular changes

- aging as chronic inflammation

- free radical theory (oxygen radicals)

- antioxidant protection (radical scavengers)

- telomere hypothesis of aging

- evolutionary theory of aging

- specific expression profiling of proteins (functional proteomics).

However, the individual life course of most living beings is modeled over time by environmental influences, genetic factors and individual lifestyle. In addition, there are explicitly uninfluenceable random factors. Aging is understood as a cellular or system-theoretical process and initially appears at the molecular level. Programs, regulations and characteristics directly related to aging are identified. Damage accumulated in the cells over time ultimately reveals the limitation of regulation (28). This process continues up the organizational hierarchy, eventually leading to death. The Werner syndrome may illustrate this process from a time-lapse perspective.

According to one of the most well-known aging theories, oxygen radicals such as ROS cause mutations on mtDNA. Therefore, mtDNA mutations accumulate over time, causing mitochondrial-mediated energy production to decrease. Adverse effects affect the heart, brain and related biological systems whose role it is to maintain health and life (24).

In normal biological aging, acquired somatic mtDNA mutations are found in post-mitotic tissues such as skeletal muscle or neurons, but also in replicative tissues, such as the colonic crypt. Such mutations have also been detected in neurodegenerative diseases (29). In contrast, some of the inherited mtDNA defects in younger people resemble diseases or disorders otherwise found in the older population: they are (senile) diabetes, hearing or visual impairments, heart or skeletal muscle weakness, movement disorders or a decline in mental abilities. In some of these tissues, but also in those which are subject to normal aging, a decrease in the activity of protein complexes that are required for energy production, for example in the respiratory chain, could be demonstrated.

The declining supply of mitochondrially generated energy via ATP appears to be the predominant cause of aging in nerves, muscles and other tissues. This makes it clear that mitochondria play a central role in the complex balance of cell processes in their energy-supplying function. Mitochondrial bioenergetic dysfunction, ultimately caused by mutations may be associated with both normal aging and age-related degenerative diseases (30) (31).

1.7 Regulation: Mitochondrial dynamics (fusion, fission)

Mitochondria have the ability to change size, shape and position simultaneously and continuously in response to cellular demand and environment (32). This phenomenon was first demonstrated by phase-contrast microscopy and later with fluorescent proteins. Depending on the cell type, the cell's physiological state or metabolic or pathogenic conditions, they fuse into a tubular network or transform into a variety of smaller fragments (33) (Fig. 11).

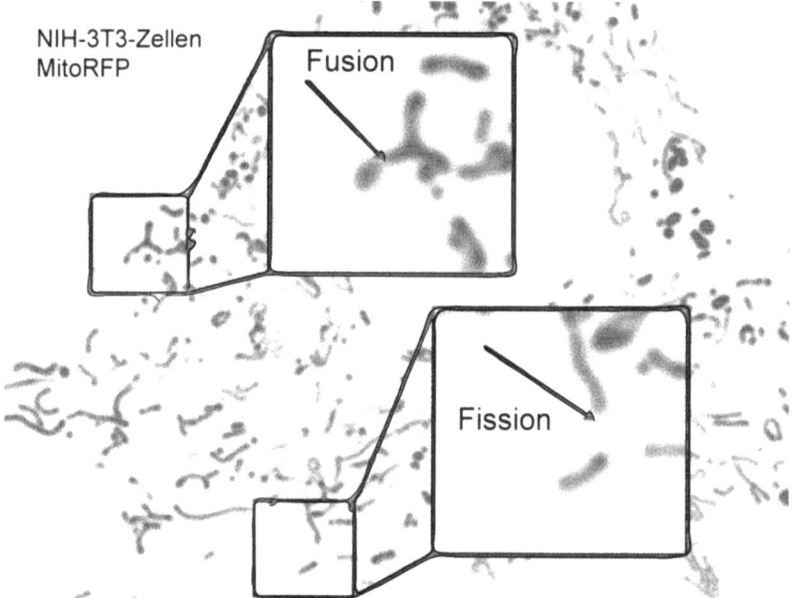

Fig. 11: Mitochondria from NIH 3T3 cells fusion and fission. Traced from an original image. See also
https://vimeo.com/107211731

Their spatial structure influences the effectiveness of energy delivery. Fibrous, interconnected network structures are capable of producing large amounts of energy, while smaller fragments are less effective. Depending on the cellular energy requirement, the functionality of the mitochondria is influenced in particular by the supply of nutrients, with the adaptation taking place dynamically via fusion and fission processes. Overnutrition also affects cell aging and function: oxidatively stressed or damaged mitochondria are fragmented and then discarded (34).

So how is a dynamic balance established between the small fragments and the effectively interconnected tubes of the mitochondria? Mathematical models point to random movements of the mitochondria along the microtubules of the cytoskeleton. In a specially designed graph model, which simulates the density of

33

microtubules and their crossing in the cell, all mitochondrial shapes found experimentally could so far be reproduced (35).

The constant reorganization of this network leads to a mixing of mitochondrial components as a prerequisite for the replenishment of oxidatively damaged mitochondrial gene products. Fusion processes are relevant for the formation of mtDNA copies for developmental biological processes such as energy transfer, intracellular signal transduction, for example by calcium or in transport processes. In Charcot-Marie-Tooth neuropathy type 2A, Charcot-Marie-Tooth neuropathy type 4A and optic atrophy type 1, a genetically justifiable fusion dysfunction seems to play a decisive role.

Alteration of these dynamics, with impairment of the fission and fusion balance and subsequent manifestation of mitochondrial dysfunction, has recently been associated with the development of neurodegenerative diseases (36) (37) (38).

In particular, there is evidence of altered fission processes in Parkinson's disease, for example through the induction of two proteins, the PTEN-induced kinase 1 (PINK1) and Parkin, which are mutated in familial forms of Parkinson's disease. In addition, mutant Huntington's protein, the disease-causing protein in Huntington's disease, alters mitochondrial morphology and dynamics. Rotenone, a pesticide and inducer of Parkinson's symptoms and Amyloid-β (Aβ) peptide, originally associated with Alzheimer's disease, initiate mitochondrial fission. And finally, fissions can also be observed in ischemic stroke or diabetic neuropathies (37).

1.8 Signaling: Senescence and Apoptosis (programmed cell death)

1.8.1 Senescence

Cellular senescence is a process that results from a variety of stresses and leads to a permanent arrest in the G0/G1-phase of the cell cycle. Such cells remain viable and metabolically active over a long period of time but are unable to enter the S-phase (39) making replication impossible. This principle, recognized in human embryonic fibroblasts (40), is accompanied by functional, cyto-morphological and metabolic changes: with an increase in volume, cells become larger, lose their original shape and develop a complex secretory phenotype (SASP = Senescence-Associated Secretory Phenotype).

SASP cells affect neighboring cells and cause tissue dysfunction over time. This process explains why senescence of once-healthy cells can promote tumor formation as well as atherosclerosis or neurodegeneration (41) (Fig.12).

Somatic cells are differentiated between replicative senescence meditated by telomere shortening (42) and an acutely activatable and telomere-independent premature senescence (43).

Telomeres are nucleoprotein structures that protect the ends of chromosomes. Unlike germ cells or stem cells, telomeres in somatic cells decrease in length with each cell division until a critical point is reached to trigger a senescence program (42). Such cells continue to live and are metabolically active, but have lost the ability to divide (44). Telomerase, a ribonucleoprotein reverse transcriptase, is responsible for specific process control and regulation to prevent genomic instability. By copying a short template sequence from its intrinsic RNA residue, telomerase synthesizes and

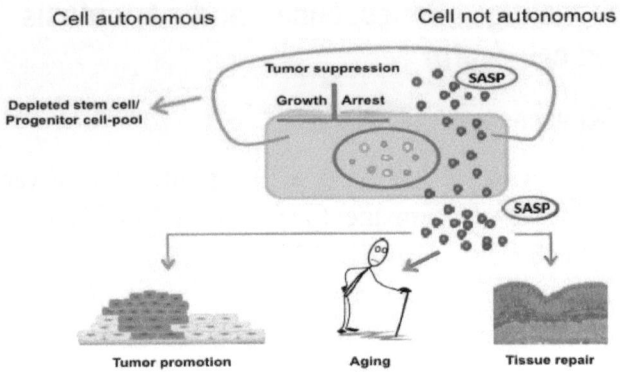

Fig. 12: Effect of the senescence-associated secretory phenotype (SASP).
Graphic: Wrobel

lengthen the telomeric DNA strand toward 5' to 3' direction at the distal end of the chromosome (45).

The other form is called premature senescence. It is activated acutely and develops independently of the telomere. In addition to stress as a potent inducer, several mitochondrial signaling pathways are involved in this mechanism. These include reactive oxygen species, mitochondrial dynamics, the electron transport chain or the calcium balance (43). In this context, a proteinopathy-induced senescence hypothesis was formulated for the genesis of Alzheimer's disease, in which highly stable misfolded protein aggregates that are not recognized as endogenous chronically activate the innate immune system. This inflammatory condition then led to premature senescence of neuronal cells. In a self-reinforcing stimulus, inflammation is perpetuated by SASP, itself a process originally triggered by inflammatory stimuli. In a neurodegenerative cascade, the senescence process of other neurons is promoted until organ failure of the brain finally occurs (46).

1.8.2 Apoptosis

Apoptosis, on the other hand, is also a mitochondrially mediated signal to trigger programmed cell death (Fig. 13). For example, when cytochrome c enters the cell's cytoplasm via a channel through the mitochondrial membrane, cell death occurs irreversibly in a set pattern (47).

From an evolutionary point of view, mitochondrially mediated apoptosis is a very old function and can be traced back to the initial stage of eukaryotic cells in metazoans. To protect the eucytic host cell, α-proteobacterium might have broken down in a symbiotic relationship in times of nutrient deficiency.

In further development, apoptosis also regulates multicellular proliferation and selects cells based on their fitness (48). This mechanism removes tissue that is not required during embryonic development, such as the separation of fingers and toes of the paddle-shaped hand attachment or of nerve cells during maturation of the nervous system, here in particular more than two thirds of all neuroblasts. Mature immune system B- or T-cells are controlled during passage in the thymus and eliminated if necessary to prevent autoimmune development. A protective function through apoptosis also exists through the elimination of virus-infected cells or those with altered genetic material. This mechanism also leads to a regular renewal of all old sensory cells, such as taste or smell, intestinal and skin cells.

Legitimate transmission of apoptotic signals is controlled by interactions with oncogenes (Bcl-2 family). If the activity is predominantly inhibitory, e.g., mediated by Bcl-2 or Bcl-xL, the functionality of the mitochondria is maintained and thus apoptosis is prevented. On the other hand, if proteins with excitatory activity such as Bax or Bak predominate, pro-apoptotic molecules are released. Cytochrome c then passes through the cytoplasm via a

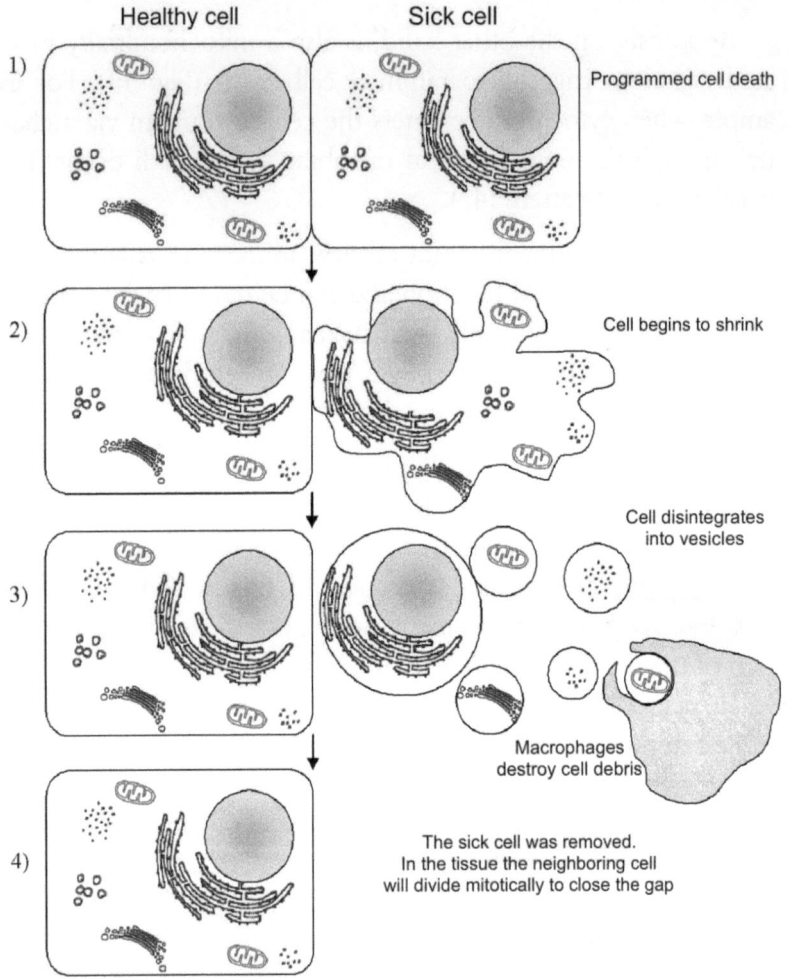

Fig. 13: Apoptotic sequence.
By H. Hoffmeister - Own work (i.e. original text: self-created), Public domain, https://commons.wikimedia.org/w/index.php?curid=7120948

channel in the mitochondrial membrane, cell death occurs irreversibly according to a fixed pattern (47): First, the cell shrinks to about 1/10 of its original size. Nucleases split the DNA into several parts, causing the cell to lose its ability to divide. Caspases separate the structural proteins such as microtubules, actin filaments and intermediate filaments, thus dissolving the cytoskeleton. The cell disintegrates into several smaller vesicles. Invading macrophages dispose of the remaining cell components. Mitosis of a neighboring cell takes the place of the destroyed one.

2 Relevant pathophysiological mechanisms

2.1 Dynamic energy metabolism

Physiological functions of neurons are essentially controlled energetically. Normally, cells obtain their ATP energy from oxidative phosphorylation. Due to age-related errors, the mitochondria are less and less able to ensure the survivability of the cell through an adequate supply of energy. The additional occurrence of oxidative stress has a neurodegenerative effect (49). In this context, an abnormal cellular bioenergetic function in Alzheimer's disease has been identified (50).

2.1.1 Astrocytes neurons lactate shuttle (ANLS)-hypothesis

Neurons consume significantly more energy than glial cells (51). Therefore, it has long been assumed that these utilize the majority of the amount of glucose. At the same time, the question arose whether they process glucose directly to meet their energy needs or whether they use some of the lactate supplied by astrocytes for this purpose (52) (53).

According to the Astrocyte Neurons Lactate Shuttle (ANLS) hypothesis, astrocytes are capable of converting glucose into lactate, which is then transferred to neurons where it is used to produce energy under aerobic conditions (Fig. 14). Glucose is taken up from the blood by the astrocytes, whose end sockets have indirect contact with the endothelial cells of the capillaries. Glucose is taken up via isoform 1 of the glucose transporter (GLUT). In the astrocytes, glucose can either be stored as glycogen or metabolized in glycolysis to pyruvate, which produces ATP. Pyruvate is subsequently metabolized to lactate by the enzyme lactate dehydrogenase isoform 5 (LDH-5) and then transferred to the neurons. For this purpose, lactate is exported from astrocytes via the mono-

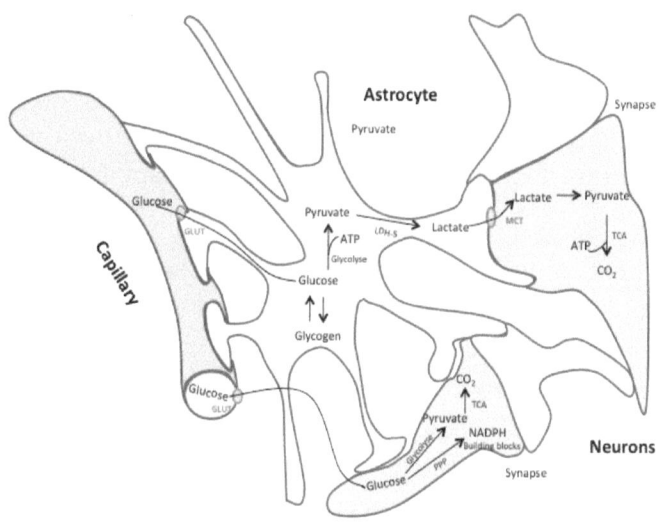

Fig. 14: Astrocyte neuron lactate shuttle hypothesis.
Graphic Wrobel

carboxylate transporters (MCT) isoforms 1 and 4 and imported into the neurons via the MCT isoform 2. In the neurons, lactate is reconverted by the enzyme lactate dehydrogenase isoform 1 (LDH-1), then metabolized in the citric acid cycle (TCA) and subsequently oxidatively phosphorylated to yield ATP. In addition to lactate, neurons also take up glucose from the parenchyma, which they import via the glucose transporter isoform 3. The absorbed glucose can either be used to generate energy by means of glycolysis, the citrate cycle and subsequent oxidative phosphorylation or in the pentose phosphate pathway (PPP) to produce building blocks for biosynthesis and the reducing agent NADPH.

The validity of this ANLS hypothesis is based on the following findings: Astrocytes have more direct access to blood-delivered nutrients including glucose. They also possess LDH isoform 5 that

41

converts pyruvate into lactate, while neurons have predominantly LDH isoform 1, which converts lactate to pyruvate. The cell-dependent expression of different isoforms of lactate transporters in astrocytes and neurons indicate a transfer of lactate from astrocytes to neurons. Lactate maintains or restores synaptic and other neuronal functions in the absence of glucose (54).

The benefit to neurons in absorbing lactate, converting it into pyruvate and processing it in the mitochondria is that it bypasses the costly process of glycolysis. This becomes important when the physiological ATP energy production decreases due to aging processes and/or the ATP energy requirement cannot be covered by regular intake. When sufficient oxygen is present, it is oxidative phosphorylation and not glycolysis that produces ATP in larger quantities. Astrocytes, on the other hand, are able to largely cover their reduced energy consumption through glycolysis. The production of energy from lactate also offers neurons the opportunity to use part of the consumed glucose not glycolytically but in the pentose phosphate pathway for the production of antioxidants and precursors for biosynthesis (55).

2.1.2 Neuroenergetic model

The neuroenergetic model (56) is based on the interaction of astrocytes and neurons, both of which use glucose as an energy source. While glucose in astrocytes is largely anaerobically metabolized to lactate and released into the extracellular milieu, pyruvate derived from glucose or lactate can be aerobically metabolized in neurons and converted to ATP energy by OxPhos (55). Neurons themselves are unable to further increase their energy production through glycolysis. When mitochondrial function is impaired, glycolysis in astrocytes is reactively upregulated, resulting in increased lactate production. If at the same time neurons upregulate their OxPhos activity, the lactate supplied by astrocytic glycolysis may be beneficial for ATP energy production (50) (57) (58). This compensatory mechanism, the upregulation of astrocytic glycolysis and mitochondrial OxPhos activity, is a complementary event that is particularly activated by mitochondria aging. The first step, first discovered in cancer metabolism is known as the Warburg effect (59), the second is the inverse Warburg effect (60).

The aging process lies between the aggregation dynamics of cellular proteins and the metabolic performance of older neurons. At the molecular level, this is driven by the increase in molecular perturbations and the concomitant decrease in enzymatic processes (61): a simultaneous decrease in chaperone and proteasome activities impairs protein aggregation and thus promotes amyloid formation. At the metabolic level, aging impacts the efficiency with which neurons adequately convert caloric energy into ATP.

In the presented neuroenergetic model, decreased efficiency is the trigger of the cascade connected with the upregulation of oxidative phosphorylation in neurons. The associated oxidative stress causes further damage to the mitochondria. The loss of neurons as a result of an insufficient energy supply leads to brain damage and thus promotes the development of dementia (60).

2.1.2.1 Side view: Warburg effect, Inverse Warburg effect

Warburg effect

In 1924, Warburg developed a hypothesis on the origin of cancer. This states that cancer cells prefer to obtain the energy they need from the anaerobic lactic acid fermentation of glucose and that oxygen is therefore not essential for cancer growth. Accordingly, tumor cells would gain their energy mainly from the fermentation of glucose and not, like healthy body cells, from cellular respiration. Common to both metabolic pathways is the build-up of glucose during glycolysis. This completes the breakdown of sugars during fermentation. The products of glycolysis are converted into lactic acid. In the course of cell respiration, however, the sugar structure is further broken down. Oxygen is only required for this complete degradation, called as the respiratory chain, which takes place in the mitochondria responsible for energy production (59) (62).

Inverse Warburg effect

The neuroenergetic model developed by Pellerin and Magistretti is based on a neuronal-astrocytic characterization of energy supply and demand in neuronal and glial cells. According to this, brain energy metabolism relies on activities of both neurons and astrocytes (63) (64).

Both cell types use glucose as an energy source. In astrocytes, a significant amount of glucose is anaerobically metabolized to lactate and released into the extracellular milieu. In neurons, on the other hand, pyruvate, derived from glucose or lactate, is metabolized aerobically, with oxidative phosphorylation being the predominant energy producer. Neurons are unable to increase energy production through glycolysis. It lacks the activities of some enzymes that promote glycolysis (65).

When some of the mitochondria in neurons become dysfunctional and thereby the energy supply decreases, compensatory measures counteract: upregulation of glycolysis in astrocytes, leading to increased lactate production and simultaneous OxPhos activities in neurons, which produce additional energy by utilizing the lactate supplied by astrocytes. Both glycolysis upregulation and OxPhos activity are two complementary methods of metabolic reprogramming.

2.2 Mitochondrial dynamics and developmental aspects.

Mutations accumulated throughout female evolutionary history have resulted in evolutionarily meaningful diversity. Newly evolved variants have allowed Homo sapiens to adapt to different environments. At the same time, this fact also provides a coherent

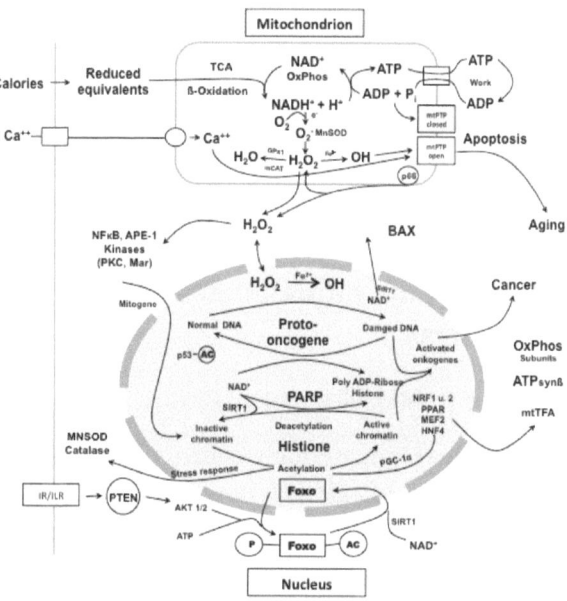

Fig. 15: Model for the effect of mitochondrial dysfunction in a cell in metabolic and degenerative diseases, aging and cancer.
Graphic Wrobel

explanation as to why modern societies tend to develop post-reproductive degenerative disease (Fig. 15):

Human ancestors were subject to very specific bioenergetic limitations. As hunters and gatherers they had to procure enough food and utilize it efficiently. The mitochondrial function adapted to these living conditions turned out to be a life-decisive factor. Such adaptive mtDNA mutations have been subjected to strict environmental control. In contrast, today in economically developed

45

societies it is possible to consume food at any time and in unlimited quantities. The energetic imbalance resulting from the discrepancy between environmentally controlled mitochondrial genetics and uncontrolled caloric intake has now led to disease-wave relevant disorders of epidemic proportions. The pathophysiology derivable from this arises from the interaction between mitochondrial energy production, ROS generation and senescent and apoptotic processes (31) (66). The utilization system responds to excess of energy via the mitochondrial dynamics. The mitochondrial network is reactively expanded by fusion processes, OxPhos is upregulated and the ATP yield is quantitatively increased. The reactive oxygen species also have a disadvantageous effect on the mtDNA due to an increased mutation rate. Ultimately, the function of a mitochondrion is impaired by an accelerated aging process (67).

2.3 Dynamics of the mtDNA-heteroplasmy and manifestation of diseases

2.3.1 Homoplasmy and Heteroplasmy

The almost exclusively maternally inherited mtDNA codes are present in large numbers of mtDNA copies in varying numbers of mitochondria in the maternal somatic cell. In addition, randomly occurring mutations in the mtDNA either occur in every copy (homoplasmy) or mutated genes and non-mutated wild types coexist in different mixing ratios (heteroplasmy) (Fig. 16).

During meiotic oocyte formation, only a small number and randomly selected mtDNA molecules from the maternal somatic cell population are transferred to the immature haploid oocytes. During the maturation process, these few molecules multiply rapidly, generating large numbers of copies.

If the mtDNA molecules transferred into the oocyte were all homoplasmic, then all subsequent copies will also be homoplasmic. On the other hand, in a heteroplasmic situation the proportions of mutant genes and wild type mtDNA can change abruptly

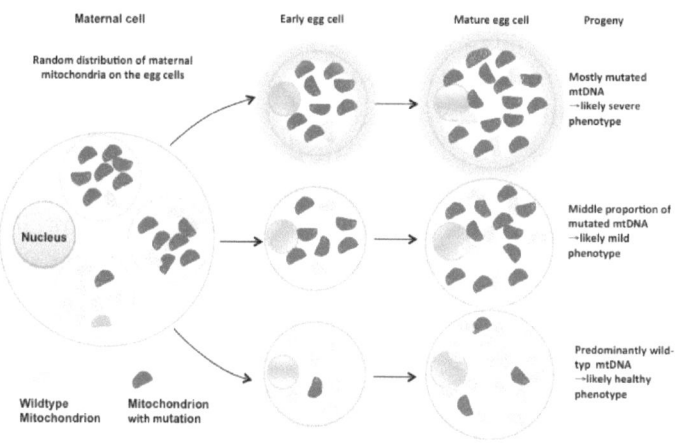

Fig. 16: Mitochondrial inheritance; the minimum disease-causing fraction (threshold effect) varies among mitochondrial mutations.
Graphic Wrobel

from generation to generation. Mothers and their offspring then show different mixing ratios in the copies (bottleneck effect) (Fig. 17).

A similar effect also exists during embryonic development. The mtDNA copies in mitochondria with different degrees of mutation mixture are also randomly distributed to daughter cells during cell division processes of the zygote.

2.3.2   Disease manifestation

Based on this mixed state alone, it is not possible to make statements about the manifestation of diseases in different tissues or organs in the heteroplasmic situation. However, it becomes more understandable why an unexpectedly large number of genes are postmitotic mutated in offspring whose mothers themselves have only a few mutations in their germ cell population or their somatic cells.

A disease that manifests itself is either attributed to an existing homoplasmy or to a changing heteroplasmy: if only a small part of the mtDNA mutates, only the performance of an organ is restricted. Further along in this process, small changes in the ratio of mutant to normal mtDNA can abruptly alter the expression of numerous genes of the nDNA with disease-causing relevance (16) (68) (69). The mutations themselves may be characterized very differently. In some, only a single nucleotide in the mtDNA is mutated (point mutation). Others also occur when larger sections

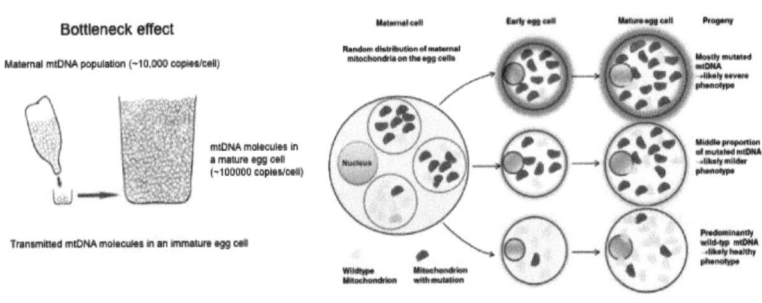

Fig. 17: Bottleneck effect of mitochondrial inheritance and consequences.
Graphic Wrobel

of mtDNA are missing (deletion) or duplicated or multiple sections are present (duplications).

Furthermore, disease-associated mutations occur not only in genes encoding proteins, but also in those encoding transferRNA (tRNA) and more rarely in genes encoding ribosomal RNA (rRNA). For example, tRNA dysfunction due to mutations impairs total protein synthesis in mitochondria (68).

Some mitochondrial diseases, such as Leber's optic neuropathy or MELAS syndrome, only manifest themselves until all mtDNA molecules have a mutation. In the heteroplasmic situation it is quite different. With little understanding of the circumstances, the proportions of mutated and non-mutated mtDNA change by

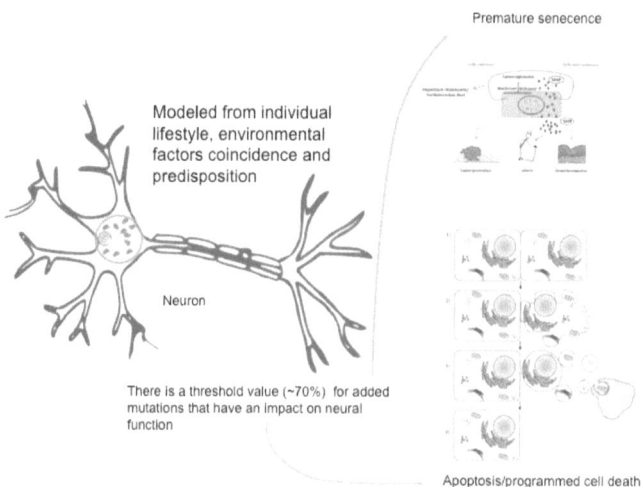

Premature senecence

Modeled from individual lifestyle, environmental factors coincidence and predisposition

Neuron

There is a threshold value (~70%) for added mutations that have an impact on neural function

Apoptosis/programmed cell death

Fig. 18: Development of the neurodegenerative disease
Graphic Wrobel

leaps and bounds from generation to generation. If a certain threshold is exceeded in the new mixture (70), a large number of very different clinical manifestations occur. Such discrete modific- ations of nuclear gene expression can best be compared to the phenomenon of a physical phase change: ice suddenly turns into water or steam when exposed to heat. Similarly, a quantitative change caused by a higher proportion of mutant mtDNA would produce a qualitative change in coordinates of nuclear gene ex- pression. The result would be a sudden, discrete change in clinical symptoms or diseases manifestations (16).

Accordingly, by no means only diseases acquired homoplasmic- ally are clinically significant, but above all those with a heteroplas- mic background, which manifest themselves as "decompensating" heteroplasmy (70) (71) (72). Finally, the dynamics of mtDNA het- eroplasmy can be conclusively explained how neurodegenerative diseases arise (72) (Fig. 18).

3 Potentially appropriate diagnostic and therapeutic procedures

According to the previous version, the extent of the mutation in the mtDNA turns out to be a health-damaging factor. Manifest diseases based on mitochondrial dysfunction are due to homoplasmy or variable heteroplasmy. If the latter decompensates, the expression of numerous genes in the nDNA changes abruptly. This gene expression profile, i.e. the pattern of gene activity at the level at which mtDNA-mutations can cause brain dysfunction is similar that seen in neurodegenerative disorders such as Alzheimer's disease (16). If this situation occurs, the specific property of the mitochondrion as an energy-supplier changes abruptly and thus also decides the fate of a neuron: it goes into an acutely activatable premature senescence or dies off through programmed cell death. Both mechanisms determine the extent to which normal brain function is impaired. In the sporadic form of Alzheimer's disease, a dysregulated or missing energy supply is therefore in the foreground. In order to be able to record the corresponding states spatially and temporally, new measurement methods are essential. This would make it necessary to develop biomarkers to adequately indicate pathological changes in the brain in a preclinical stage.

3.1 Diagnostic options

3.1.1 Further development of optical information-based biomarkers

Understanding the physiology in health or disease states requires quantitative analysis of ion and metabolite dynamics with subcellular resolution in vivo to analyze metabolic processes. Recent developments in the field of optical imaging enable the visualization of tissue microstructures and thus help to quantitatively depict disease-specific endogenous and exogenous substances. Such technologies are suitable for non-invasive and objective diagnostics and for monitoring-initiated therapies (73).

For example, genetically encoded Förster resonance energy transfer (FRET) sensors are used for real-time in-vivo detection of metabolites. FRET sensor proteins, like those for glucose, can be genetically targeted to any cell compartment or even subdomains, like a membrane surface, by adding signaling sequences or fusing the sensors to specific proteins. These sensors are used for analyses in single mammalian cells in culture, tissues and intact organisms. Applications include gene detection, high-throughput drug screening and systematic analysis of regulatory networks. Quantitative analyses obtained using FRET sensors for glucose or other ions and metabolites provide valuable data for modeling fluxes such as the monitoring glucose levels in the cytosol of mammalian cell cultures. In principle, such protocols are also applicable for other ions and metabolites as well as for analyzes in other organisms, such as bacteria, yeasts or intact plants (74) (75).

In brain tissue, some energy metabolites have turnover times ranging from milliseconds to seconds and are rapidly exchanged between cells and within cells. Until recently, these rapid metabolic events have not been accessible because standard isotopic techniques require the use of cell populations and/or involve integration times of minutes. Thanks to fluorescent probes and now available genetically encoded optical nanosensors, this technology is set in to monitor levels of metabolites in real-time and in single cells. In combination with ad hoc inhibitor-stop protocols, these probes have demonstrated a key role for potassium K^+ in the acute stimulation of astrocytic glycolysis through synaptic activity. The Warburg effect could also be reproduced in individual cancer cells. Genetically encoded nanosensors currently exist for glucose, lactate, NADH and ATP and other metabolite nanosensors will soon be available. These optical tools, together with improved expression systems and in-vivo imaging, enable accurate analysis of cellular metabolism in different states (76) (77).

Lactate is transferred between and within cells and plays metabolic and signaling roles in healthy tissues. As a harbinger of altered metabolism, lactate is also involved in pathogenesis, for example in neurodegeneration or carcinogenesis. So, in the presence of oxygen, tumor cells produce high levels of lactate, a phenomenon known as the Warburg effect. This effect has now been confirmed in vivo with a genetically encoded FRET-based nanosensor for lactate by measuring its concentration and flux in single mammalian cells (78).

3.1.1.1 Energy metabolism

Measuring OxPhos activity is a good way to identify dysregulations in energy metabolism. Using genetically encoded fluorescence biosensors, it is possible to spatially resolve the presence of various metabolites in living cells continuously, non-invasively and in real-time (76) (79).

The measurement signal of many of these biosensors is based on a change in the intensity of a Förster resonance energy transfer (FRET). Typical FRET-based biosensors consist of E. coli periplasmic binding domains to which c-terminal and n-terminal color variants of green-fluorescent-protein (GFP) have been fused. Due to a conformational change in protein structure in binding domains that occurs upon ligand binding, the spatial distance and orientation of the fluorescent proteins relative to each other change. As a result, there is a change in the FRET-signal intensity, which can be interpreted as a direct indication of the presence of the ligand. For example, lactate plays a metabolic and signaling role in healthy tissues. Using a genetically encoded FRET-based nanosensor, the Warburg effect could be confirmed by measuring lactate concentration and lactate flux in single mammalian cells in vivo (78). Accordingly, this method is suitable to measure OxPhos activity as a biomarker to detect neurodegeneration. Such nanosensors are available for glucose, lactate, NADH and ATP (79).

3.1.1.2 Mitochondrial redox marker

Imbalances in ROS homeostasis promote oxidative stress, included an increased risk of mutations in nuclear and mitochondrial DNA (27) (80). Numerous techniques, assays and biomarkers are used to predict the level of oxidative stress by measuring reactive oxygen species (ROS) and nitrogen species (RNS). In this way, electron paramagnetic resonance spectroscopy can be performed to assess the strengths and limitations of different ROS or RNS measurement methods (81).

The glutathione system serves a mitochondrial redox-biomarker. With improved analytical techniques in virtually any tissue sample or with analytical imaging techniques, such as HMPAO SPECT, it is possible to estimate redox imbalance via glutathione metabolites (82).

3.1.1.3 NADH/FAD

Early detection of mitochondrial and metabolic abnormalities is an essential step to make timely diagnoses and design therapeutic interventions effectively. Reduced nicotinamide adenine dinucleotide (NADH) and flavin adenine dinucleotide (FAD) are relevant to a broad spectrum of cellular redox reactions and allow measurements of metabolic status. NADH and FAD are inherently fluorescent and are excited at different wavelengths to produce complementary imaging (83).

With the highly sensitive, genetically encoded fluorescence sensor SoNar (sensor of NAD(H) redox) it is possible to monitor the NAD^+/NADH redox state in living cells and in vivo. Binding to either NAD^+ or NADH affects their fluorescent properties (84). This biosensor is perfectly suited to detect disturbances in energy metabolism in real-time.

Intracellular NADH and FAD are potential biomarkers for recording metabolic and mitochondrial activities (83).

3.1.1.4 Mitochondrial dynamics

Mitochondrial morphology varies in cell types and tissues and changes rapidly in response to external stimuli and nutrient status (38) (85) (86) via fusion and fission processes. Inappropriate fission leads to fragmentation of mitochondria and is associated with metabolic dysfunction and disease. On the other hand, improper fusion results in a hyperfused network that tends to counteract metabolic dysfunction, maintain cell integrity and protect against autophagy (86). By identifying several fusion and fission regulators such as Drp1, OPA1 or mitofusins, deeper insights have been gained due to the pathogenesis of neurodegenerative diseases associated with impaired mitochondrial dynamics (85) (87).

Optical imaging methods are used for microstructural tissue mapping of disease-specific endogenous and exogenous substances, suitable for non-invasive diagnostics and for initiated therapies. Appropriate methods include spectroscopic techniques (73). For example, based on photothermal optical coherence microscopy and using a novel surface functionalization of gold nanoparticles, the mitochondrial dynamics of living HeLa cells are monitored with a 3D time-lapse imaging technique. To quantify them, temporal autocorrelation analysis is combined with a classic diffusion mode. The representation of the results in 3D maps demonstrates the heterogeneity of the diffusion parameters over the entire cell volume (88). Therefore, image-based methods are suitable as biomarkers for mitochondrial phenotyping (89).

3.1.2 Biomarkers to detect neuronal senescence and apoptosis

3.1.2.1 Senescence

Cellular senescence describes the cessation of growth in aging cells and is found in glia and neurons in Alzheimer's disease. Included are phenotypes associated with cellular senescence such as cytokines, epigenetic regulation and protein expression (90) (Fig. 19).

Senescent cells are part of a unique mechanism of time-dependent tissue dysfunction. They negatively affect neighboring cells that originate from an altered so-called senescence-associated secretory phenotype (SASP). This disadvantageously promotes senescence of healthy cells or tumor formation, as well as atherosclerosis or neurodegeneration. In the case of interventions, e.g., the removal of senescent cells, a reliable biomarker is essential for understanding aging processes (91).

For example, one of the best characterized and simplified methods of measuring senescence in vitro and in vivo is the β-galactosidase (β-Gal) assay, which measures β-Gal activity. This is the activity expressed by senescent cells detectable by immunohistochemistry at pH 6.0. β-Gal is only detectable in senescent cells and not in presenescent or quiescent fibroblasts or keratinocytes, making it a reliable marker for detecting senescent cells in multiple organisms and conditions. In this way, senescence-associated β-Gal (SA-β-Gal) can be reliably detected in skin samples from human donors as a function of age. The SA-β-Gal protocol involves

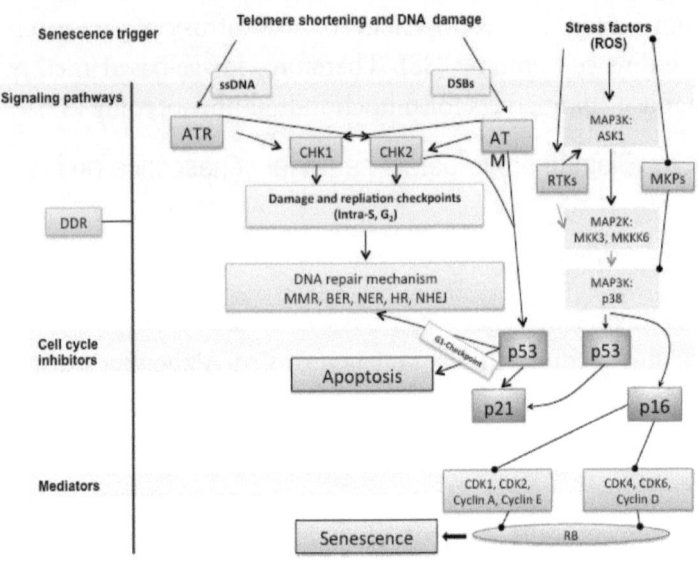

Fig. 19: Graphical representation of two senescence signaling cascades: Triggers (telomere shortening/DNA damage and stress factors/ROS) activate cell cycle inhibitors that induce senescence via mediators.
Graphic Wrobel

staining cells or tissues with X-Gal (5-bromo-4-chloroindoly-β-D-galactoside or another fluorescent analogue such as FDG), a chromogenic substrate of β-Gal. X-Gal is cleaved by β-Gal resulting in an insoluble blue dye. SA-β-Gal has been identified as a senescent marker in a replicative senescence protocol or by senescence-induced methods using DNA-damaging agents, oncogenic signaling or overexpression of tumor suppressors such as p16 and ARF (92).

Age-dependent neurons also develop a senescence-like phenotype that starts in the lysosomal part and simultaneously contents lysosomal β-galactosidase (93). A pronounced induction of SA-β-gal activity in the hippocampus has been observed experimentally in vivo (94). Senescence-associated β-galactosidase (SA-β-gal) may be used as a biomarker to identify neuronal senescence.

Telomere shortening has been identified as a stress-response phenomenon. In the peripheral blood cells of people with Alzheimer's disease, shorter telomeres were found than in age-matched controls. It has also been observed that fibroblasts in the sporadic form of Alzheimer's disease specifically have an abnormal and detectable conformational state of the mutant-like senescence-marker p53, which allows differentiation of appropriate patients (95). Peripheral blood cells from affected individuals are also more sensitive to apoptosis. An increased rate of apoptosis in $CD4^+$-T cells as well as in natural killer cells accompanied by an increased expression of the anti-apoptotic protein B-cell lymphoma 2 (Bcl-2), the antioxidant enzyme superoxide dismutase 1 (SOD1) and various caspase subtypes 17).

3.1.2.2 Apoptosis/Programmed cell death

Among other things, apoptosis is also a mitochondrial-mediated signal for triggering programmed cell death (Fig. 20). In addition to the apoptotic form of programmed cell death, there is also an autophagy-mediated form (96) (97). In Alzheimer's disease, this process is modulated in a variety of ways, for example by cell surface receptors, caspases, mitochondrial factors or p53 (98).

In this context, suitable biomarkers are presenilin proteins (PSEN1, PSEN2) (3), but also the anti-apoptotic protein Bcl-2, the antioxidant enzyme superoxide dismutase 1 (SOD1) or various subtypes of caspases (17) (99).

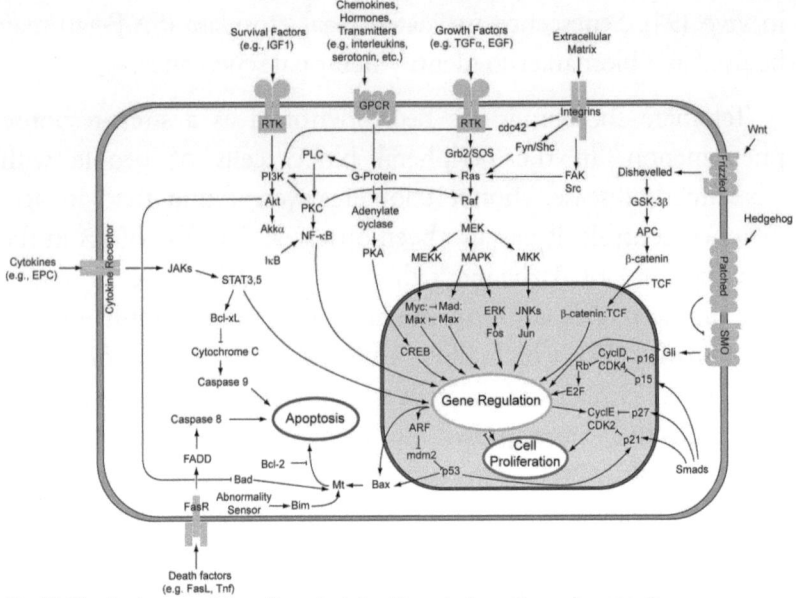

Fig. 20: Simplified representation of important signal transduction pathways in mammals.
By Roadnottaken from the English Wikipedia, CC BY-SA 3.0, https://commons.wikimedia.org/w/index.php?curid=2163484

3.2 Therapeutic options

Alzheimer's patients currently have four synthetically produced active ingredients available: the three acetylcholinesterase inhibitors donepezil, rivastigmine and galantamine and the NMDA antagonist memantine. They can delay mental decline, alleviate some of the symptoms and slightly improve daily functioning (100). Non-pharmacologic treatments encompass a range of therapeutic and individualized treatment options. Molecular biological and genetic or epigenetic therapeutic strategies aim, among others things, at the use of antibodies or active and passive immunization or signaling in the immune system (101). A breakthrough has not yet happened (11).

3.2.1   Multimodal therapy approaches

It is estimated that one third of Alzheimer's diseases worldwide are due to preventable risk factors such as morbid obesity, diabetes mellitus, hypertension, physical inactivity, smoking and depression (102).

Against this background, multimodal approaches were reviewed suggesting that the decline in cognitive performance in older people can be halted by healthy diet or exercise and cognitive training in combination with constant control of vascular risk parameters (Finnish Geriatric Intervention Study to Prevent Cognitive Impairment and Disability). Indeed, such intervention strategies could reduce the risk of age-related neurodegeneration (103) (104). Another approach to maintaining brain health relies on a combination of lifestyle modification and specific anti-Alzheimer's therapies (105) (106). But the individual attitude towards life may also have a positive influence on this (107). A similar strategy is followed in the concept of mitohormesis through appropriate nutrition and sufficient exercise. A therapeutic interaction with reactive oxygen species has been postulated (108).

The bioenergetic model used to explain Alzheimer's disease focusses on energy metabolism. Suitable therapeutics agents would specifically intervene in the relevant processes such as glucose metabolism or substrate supply. Other intervention strategies target ROS damage or removal of damaged mitochondria burdened by apoptosis or mitophagy (109). However, most of these therapeutic approaches are still in the experimental stage.

3.2.2   Metabolic interventions

The neuronal microenvironment is altered to affect cellular metabolism. Lactate produced and mediated by astrocytes is a potential energy source for neurons (110) and is involved in brain glucose metabolism via neuron-lactate shuttles. Metabolic therapy would target this process (111). Medium chain triglycerides are used as part of a ketogenic diet effective in reducing epileptic episodes. The brain health benefits of medium-chain fatty acids can be thought of as the extra energy intake that comes from stimulating liver ketogenesis. Basically, the astrocyte-neuron-lactate and ketone body shuttle system supplies neighboring neurons in the form of lactate or ketone bodies (112).

3.2.3 Antioxidant therapy

Antioxidants are endogenous or exogenous mostly low-molecular substances that either reduce or neutralize the formation of free radicals. Antioxidants can be fat-soluble or water-soluble, differ in their ability to cross the blood-brain barrier, are membrane-soluble or detoxify peroxides. Appropriate therapies have shown only limited success to date (27).

3.2.4 Mitochondrial dynamics

Mitochondria are highly dynamic organelles that continuously fuse, fission and transport. Morphology, number and function are regulated and controlled by mitochondrial dynamics (Fig. 21) (Fig.22). In principle, new therapeutic strategies can be derived from this (87) (113).

(A) Drp1 in the cytosol is recruited by multiple receptor proteins in the mitochondria outer membrane and oligomerized into ring-like structures. This partially constricts the mitochondrial membrane. Another dynamin-like protein, dynamin 2 (Dyn2), binds and further constricts the mitochondrial membrane to allow lipid fusion and organelle

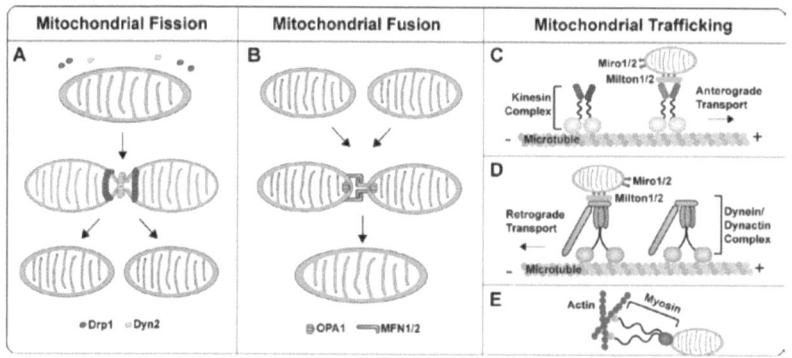

F

ig. 21: Schematic representation of mitochondrial dynamics in mammalian cells. Abnormalitis of Mitochondrial Dynamics in Neurodegenerative Diseases.
By Ju Gao 1, Luwen Wang 1, Jingyi Liu 1, Fei Xie 1, Bo Su 2 and Xinglong Wang. Antioxidants 2017, 6(2), 25 (CC BY 4.0).

division. (B) The mitochondrial fusion process requires two steps: outer and inner membrane fusion. Outer membrane fusion is mediated by interactions of coiled-coil domains of Mfn1 and Mfn2 to form either homo-oligomeric or hetero-oligomeric membrane-tethering complexes. OPA1 is involved in the formation of cristae junctions and in inner membrane fusion. (C,D) The anterograde motor kinesin-1 and retrograde motor dynein/dynactin complexes interact directly with milton and miro on mitochondria to control their movement along the microtu-

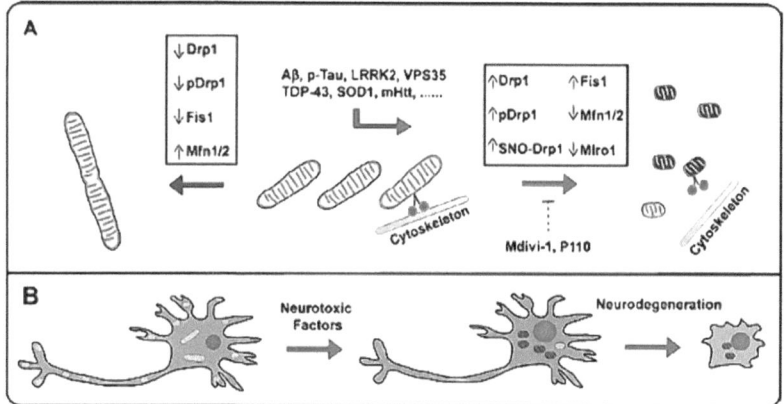

Fig. 22: Abnormalities of Mitochondrial Dynamics in Neurodegenerative Diseases.
By Ju Gao 1, Luwen Wang 1, Jingyi Liu 1, Fei Xie 1, Bo Su 2 and Xinglong Wang. Antioxidants 2017, 6(2), 25 (CC BY 4.0).

bules. (E) Actin motors are associated with mitochondria to facilitate short-distant movement along the filament.

(A) Mitochondrial fragmentation is a common factor in neurodegeneration resulting in impaired mitochondrial function and increased cell death. Disease-associated proteins such as phosphorylated tau, Aβ, LRRK2 G2019S, SOD1 G93A and Htt mutants disrupt mitochondrial dynamics, including fusion, fission and transport leading to mitochondrial dysfunction. Manipulation of mitochondrial dynamics through genetic or chemical approaches is arguably a useful strategy for restoring mitochondrial function and promoting neuronal survival.

(B) Mitochondrial dynamic abnormalities impair mitochondrial transport and proper localization, leading to mitochondrial depletion in neurites and synapses and eventual neuronal death.

3.2.5 Homoplasmy and Heteroplasmy, CrisprCas9 technology and gene replacement therapy

In the maternal somatic cell, non-mutant wild types and mutations are differentially distributed in mtDNA copies during meiotic oocyte formation and during embryonic development. In principle, it is possible to influence mutations in the mtDNA. All therapeutic approaches derived from this are at an experimental stage.

There are two new approaches to preventing and treating mitochondrial diseases: reducing mutant mitochondrial load during gene replacement therapy. And applying the principles of bacterial immune function via CrisprCas9 technology to target specific sequences of mutant DNA for removal (114). Mitochondrial replacement therapy is a promising technique to prevent transmission of a higher mutant mitochondrial load. However, it is ethically controversial because donor embryo is used to transplant nuclear DNA. After reconstitution of the oocytes, spindles are inserted into the cytoplasm of the nucleated donor oocytes. It is a novel technology to prevent mtDNA transfer from oocytes to preimplantation embryos (115).

4 New view on the Neurodegeneration of the sporadic form of Alzheimer's disease

4.1 Evolutionary environmental interactions

The development of bioenergetic disorders of cell function has a complex background. The archaic structures inherited in each cell have been exposed to competition in an ever-changing environment from the start. Crucial to this evolutionary process was the development of eucytes from LUCA and mitochondria as part of endosymbiosis. The eukaryotic cells that evolved became capable of enhanced internal energy production, allowing them to process, store and use information effectively.

The interaction with the environment required for the normal bioenergetic function of a cell relates to the formation and utilization of energy products such as glucose. It is formed from carbon dioxide CO_2 and water H_2O. With solar emitted photons, the photosynthetic process releases oxygen O_2 into the environment. Glucose is utilized in the mitochondrial respiratory chain by a fractionated oxyhydrogen reaction. The oxygen O_2 required for this reaches the intracellular space through inspiration from the environment. As a universal principle, energy is formed in the structure of ATP while CO_2 is released into the environment through exhalation.

Relevant environmental interactions of Homo sapiens were inevitably geared towards food intake and primarily aimed at the optimal utilization of energy-rich substrates. The adverse circumstances of our human ancestors as hunters and gatherers meet today a society with an abundance of food. The "old" environmentally controlled mitochondrial genetics designed for efficient food utilization are overridden by the "modern" uncontrolled caloric intake.

The mitochondrial network increasingly reacts to this excess energy with fusion processes. The reactively upregulated oxidative phosphorylation then quantitatively raises the ATP yield. At the same time, however, the growth in reactive oxygen species has an adverse effect on the mtDNA due to an enhanced mutation rate. Ultimately, the function of a mitochondrion is impaired by an accelerated aging process.

4.2   Inverse Warburg effect

The interaction of astrocytes and neurons, both of which use glucose as an energy source, is sufficiently well explained in the neuroenergetic model (Fig. 14). While glucose in the astrocytes is largely metabolized anaerobically to lactate and released into the extracellular milieu, glucose or lactate produced from pyruvate is metabolized aerobically and converted into ATP energy by Ox-Phos. Neurons themselves are unable to further increase their energy production through glycolysis. When mitochondrial function is impaired, glycolysis in astrocytes is reactively upregulated resulting in increased lactate production. If, at the same time, neurons upregulate their OxPhos activity, the lactate supplied from astrocytic glycolysis can be used to produce ATP energy. This compensatory mechanism, the upregulation of astrocytic glycolysis and mitochondrial OxPhos activity, is a complementary event that is particularly activated during mitochondria aging.

4.3   Consequences of mtDNA-mutations: Senescence and programmed cell death

The extent of existing mutations in the mtDNA proves to be harmful to health. The manifestation of the disease can be traced back to mitochondrial dysfunction. It is attributed to either existing homoplasmy or altered heteroplasmy. If the latter decompensates, the expression of numerous genes in the nDNA change abruptly. This gene expression profile, i.e., the pattern of gene activity at the level at which mtDNA-mutations cause brain dysfunction resembles the profile found in neurodegenerative disorders such as Alzheimer's disease (16). If this situation occurs, the specific property of the mitochondrion as an energy-supplier changes abruptly and thus also decides the fate of a neuron: it undergoes an acutely activated premature senescence or dies off as a result of programmed cell death. During disposal, the free space is filled by proliferating glia. The extent of both mechanisms determines the extent of impairment of normal brain function.

4.4 Consequences of disturbed protein quality control

In the sporadic form of Alzheimer's disease, ß-amyloid plays a rather subordinate role depending on the disease. Age and bioenergetic mitochondrial dysfunction also have a negative effect on the function of the chaperones. They usually check the correct folding of proteins, such as ß-amyloid (Aß) as a protein fragment of the amyloid precursor protein (APP). When properly folded, the protein is released from the endoplasmic reticulum by vesicles. With decreasing protein quality control mediated by chaperones, the number of misfolded proteins that cannot be physiologically degraded by secretases increases. Their removal is therefore restricted. Finally, such intracellularly deposited aggregates (116) (117) (118) also impede electron transport in the respiratory chain and thus mitochondrial function (119).

4.5 Energetic-genetic interrelationship

The preceding explanation makes it clear why the interplay of energetic and genetic components is the determining factor. Genetic and environmental stressors cause altered mitochondrial dynamics and thus mitochondrial dysfunction (38). Against an evolutionarily justifiable metabolic background, it is understandable why this disease increases exponentially with age and why a therapy aimed solely at the genetic component with removal of the amyloid (2) is not very promising. The sporadic form of Alzheimer's disease is primarily due to a normal aging process that is randomly modeled by individual lifestyle, environmental factors and predisposition.

4.6   Brain plasticity

Due to the plasticity of the brain with a large reserve capacity, which in principle can be tapped through intensive intellectual activity (120) (121), there is a wide spectrum of clinical manifestations. The decisive factor here is the density of the existing synapses in the brain and not the extent of the extracellular and intracellular amyloid deposits (122) (123). For example, in the very early stages of Alzheimer's disease, memory is impaired, subtly related to synaptic dysfunction in the hippocampal region that is detectable even before neuronal degeneration. Despite the complexity of the etiology of this disease, synaptic failure due to reduced synaptic density, synaptic transmission or lack of synaptic plasticity is a major feature of this disease (122).

4.7   Healthy and pathological aging

In healthy aging patients, there is a functional balance between damaged and intact mitochondria with little initial impairment of brain performance (60). In contrast, numerous epidemiological studies (124) indicate that the transition to pathological aging occurs in many people as a result of an acute event such as a stroke, myocardial infarction, traumatic brain injury, partner loss or other life-changing events (125) (126) (127) (128) (129) (130).

4.8   Result and conclusions

The aim of all efforts should be to maintain the health balance in healthy aging Alzheimer's sufferers and, if possible, to restore a disturbed one. Lifelong prevention, which includes diet, physical cognitive training and lifestyle modification is the best treatment option. Against the background of the currently very limited drug therapy options, more attention should be paid to the extent to which therapeutic interventions in the metabolic and energy processes of the brain are possible.

In summary, the onset of the sporadic form of Alzheimer's disease is primarily due to normal aging, followed by a combination of pure and deterministic chance, influenced by environmental factors and predisposition. Fate decides whether such an exposed person falls ill.

From the chain of arguments presented, it can finally be deduced how dysfunctional mitochondria may actually be at the top of the cascade of the sporadic form of Alzheimer's disease. In contrast, the reductionist approaches of purely molecular biological and genetic processes do not make a satisfactory contribution to the understanding the development of this form of the disease. Even if this is now better understood pathoetiogenetically, the question remains whether this finding has solved a possible chicken-egg problem. So what exactly is behind this disease, what is its secret?

The high efficiency in energy utilization and ATP energy production mediated by mitochondria cannot be explained in classical biophysical or chemical terms. Neither is the fundamental development of mutations at the mtDNA level, which ultimately renders mitochondria inoperable. What happens energetically at the subatomic level cannot be explained solely according to the principles of classical thermodynamics. And finally, there is also the question of the original principle of life.

According to recent findings, some kind of elementary information could be behind the secret. If you follow quantum information theory, timeless, spaceless and meaningless information condenses into energy or matter via photons that make up the 4-dimensional world we know. Against this background at least the properties and processes of the inanimate can be described in terms of quantum physics, but the animate requires a different approach.

5 A different view of the origin of the sporadic form of Alzheimer's disease: Quantum biological background

5.1 From biological quantum physics to quantum biology

The properties and interactions of matter particles or waves known from quantum mechanics can be demonstrated experimentally at the subatomic level, mostly at temperatures close to absolute zero. The most important process at the elementary level is fluctuation. Fluctuation clearly means the emergence of "something" from "nothing" without regularity, i.e., purely by chance. Mathematically and physically, this process is best to describe as the superposition of waves and of probabilities (=coherence) (131). By another process, this time through information-processing (=measurement process), the superposition of waves is removed (=decoherence). At that moment, the indefinite abstract becomes something concrete: it is the inanimate matter that we are able to comprehend, the properties of which are largely deciphered in classical physics.

In contrast, living beings and their evolutionary history are the subject of scientific study through biology. In the evolutionary context, parallels between ontogeny and phylogeny (132) initially led to the realization that there are causal relationships between ontogenetic and evolutionary processes (133). However, the true mechanisms for generating genetic variability were only uncovered with knowledge from genetics (134) and are summarized in population genetics:

▤ Mutation is an undirected search process and generates

70

variants and alternatives.

- ▤ Through the recombination of long nucleotide chains, genetic information is exchanged between the homologous chromosomes of the parent generation, i.e., gene combinations that have already been tested are remixed in the sense of an optimization process.
- ▤ Above all, selection as a deterministic process should determine the direction of movement of evolution.

Evolution can be viewed as a feedback-driven process. Living beings not only adapt to their environment, but also change the habitat they occupy by their mere existence. In this way, according to Verhulst, the developmental dynamics of a population with limited habitat is describable mathematically as follows:

$$x_{n+1} = r \, x \, n - r \, x_n^2$$

The selection follows a non-linear dynamic and is therefore a non-deterministic, chaotic process: there is no predictable, but a seriously different order, generated by random, minor changes in the boundary condition. Accordingly, *non-deterministic chaos* arises from unpredictable changes in the state of objective random factors. The unpredictability of a *deterministic chaos*, on the other hand, does not result from simple coincidences, but solely from the inherent dynamics of such systems.

The unpredictability of biological systems, such as the interaction of the cells of an individual or the development of organs, results on the one hand from the abundance of influencing factors and on the other hand from the structure-related non-measurability of certain elementary states, quite in analogy to Heisenberg's uncertainty principle (135).

In general, natural phenomena follow a Gaussian distribution. This is an ideal form of a commonly observed frequency distribution in biological, psychological and sociological variables (Fig. 23).

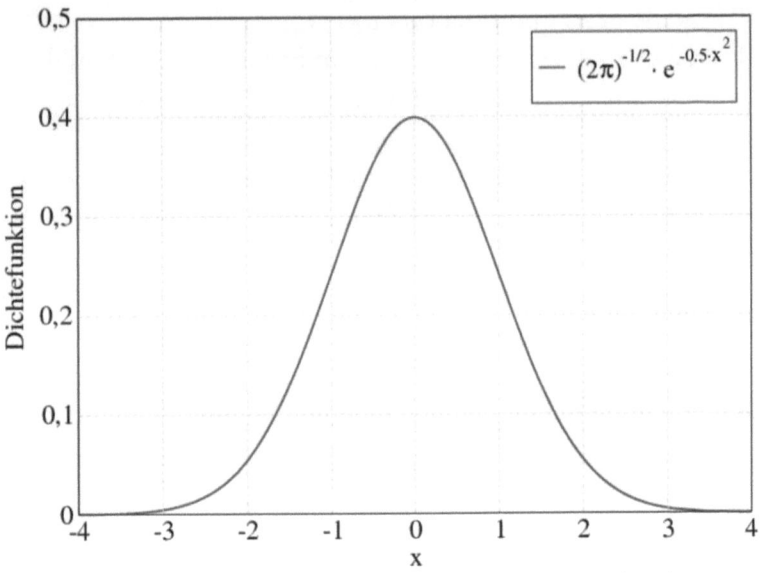

Fig. 23: Density function of the standard normal distribution (Gaussian normal distribution).

Intermediate values are most common, extreme characteristics are rarer. A normal distribution is expected when a variable is influenced by numerous factors that are independent and additive.

A pillar of quantum physics that is also valid in biology is based on the knowledge that the position and momentum of a particle cannot, in principle, be determined with any degree of precision at the same time. Simultaneous determining of position and momentum of a particle is only possible if a certain degree of uncertainty is accepted for both quantities. There is a relationship between the quantities known as the Heisenberg uncertainty principle:

$$\Delta x \; \Delta p \geq \hbar/2 = h/4 \, \pi$$

Consequently, the position and momentum of a quantum object cannot be determined simultaneously with any degree of accuracy.

Also, in contrast to the Platonic world view, nature is presented as an actually imperfect geometry solely for the purpose of creating the greatest possible variety of forms. As a self-similar phenomenon, it expresses itself as a fractal (136): repetitive basic patterns in an alternation between regularity and irregularity and broken non-integer dimension.

However, how things behave differently and weirdly with quantum physics will be made clear in the following: the term "non-locality" (137) means space and timelessness. In this state, subatomic structures can only be understood with a certain probability and show different properties at each point in time. When the system is entangled, a certain kind of information is transmitted faster than the speed of light. This means that regardless of local occurrences and phenomena in our world, there is another hitherto inaccessible one that is immediate and instantaneous, meaning that it is able to communicate faster than the speed of light. Or, for example, insurmountable potential barriers at the subatomic level are penetrated via a certain mechanism of coherent tunneling of electrons or protons. What is special, however, is the measurement process, which is demonstrated in the double-slit experiment. As a result, the behavior of particles or systems is directly influenced solely by the observation conditions. Science has not even begun to understand what exactly is behind these properties and processes. At best, an attribution would succeed if one were allowed to associate this strange behavior with "some kind of consciousness". In the semantically common language, this term is fundamentally different from that of consciousness and is best understood as information-processing. A detailed description of the facts would go beyond the scope of this work. *In order to avoid misunderstandings, the term "awareness" is used the following in a paraphrased manner.*

Quantum biology has evolved from biophysics and quantum physics (138) (139) (140) (141) and deals with the experimental and theoretical investigation of non-trivial quantum phenomena in biological systems (142). It addresses corresponding phenomena, such as those that occur in the interaction of photons with living cells of an organism. The energetic processes and changes in the area of atoms and molecules are examined. In living nature, the phenomena of quantum physics can be demonstrated primarily at normal temperatures.

5.2   Physical reality and realness

According to the more recent philosophy of science and modern psychology, two terms that were once considered synonymous have turned out to be opposites: *the set of all objectively true statements is called reality, regardless of whether they are known or even recognizable to an individual person or humanity as a whole. Realness, on the other hand, is the set of statements that an individual or group of people believe to be true.*

In this context, a real physical entity can best be derived as a description of a closed system with full applicability of the law of conservation of energy:

- a 4-dimensional (metric) *reality*,
- and at the same time a spaceless and timeless (metric-free) *realness*,
- information-processing (= physical measuring process). This creates interactions within the system.
- constant energy in a closed system.

In summary, this leads to the following conclusion:

- When work is done in metric reality, entropy is generated.
- In the temporal context, the system reaches a maximum with an increasing entropy, which physically means its heat death.
- To avoid this condition, entropy must be transferred from metric reality to metric-free realness.
- The transfer to the metric-free realness is possible through information-processing.
- In the metric-free realness something emerges that can be described semantically as an information store.
- In the information store of the metric-free realness there is a type of information that is equivalent to energy or matter called "elementary information". If that type of information had any other property, the law of conservation of energy would be violated.
- In the metric-free realness, elementary information is a concrete part of the system, but from the point of view of metric reality it is abstract.
- Equivalent matter or energy arises from elementary information through information-processing.
- Entropy must also be equivalent to what is physically generated by information-processing. Otherwise, the law of conservation of energy would also be violated.

▤ Any performance of physical work in the metric realness is always associated with information-processing.

Regardless of the local appearances and phenomena of reality according to the above definition, a metrically inaccessible realness with direct and instantaneous interaction can be derived. Together it is a true physical entity.

With the help of this view, it is possible to formulate questions from which further knowledge can be gained by means of scientific empirical methods.

The fact that enzymes act in the midst of thermodynamically highly active cells suggests the development of special abilities in living structures. As has now been experimentally proven, enzymes are able to prevent the decoherence of the interacting system for a sufficiently long time. Somehow they claim quantum physical tunneling effects for their specific functions. What is particularly remarkable is how they do this

▤ active
▤ targeted
▤ needs-based.

Quite obviously enzymes interact on different levels of reality. In contrast to pure chance with condensation of photons through fluctuation and decoherence, they are capable of an interactive process and control it in a targeted and needs-based manner.

5.3 From statistical-physical to elementary information: Bit and Qubit

In the 4-dimensional world, animals and plants appear as self-organizing, dissipative and open non-equilibrium systems (143) functioning as living space-time constructs. Life and development processes follow non-linear dynamics and strive for disorder. Only then do tendencies towards heterogeneity, diversification, differentiation and instability evolve. Living beings embody systems with very high potential energies and at the same time represent a high degree of order, protected by self-organization against disruption tendencies.

5.3.1 Relationship between statistical information and entropy

Specific aspects of life and development processes can be studied using statistical Boltzmann-entropy (a) and Shannon-information (b).

a.) Definition of the entropy S as logarithm of the probability

p (k_B = Boltzmann constant 1.381 10^{-23} J/K):

$$S = k_B \log p$$

Entropy can thus be used sensibly in many contexts as a statistically defined quantity.

b.) The information content of a character x with an occurrence probability Px is defined as:

$$I(p_x) = \log_a \left(\frac{1}{p_x} \right) = -\log_a(p_x)$$

a corresponds to the power of an alphabet, i.e., the number of possible states of a message source.

The information content I_{ges} of a sequence of n statistically independent events with probabilities of occurrence of:

$I(p1)$, $I(p2)$, ..., $I(pn)$ *is* then calculated from:

$$I_{ges} = I(p_1) + I(p_2) + I(p_3) + \ldots + I(p_n) = \sum_{k=1}^{n} I(p_k)$$

One of the key experiments to identify connections between energy and information can be presented as follows (Fig 24):

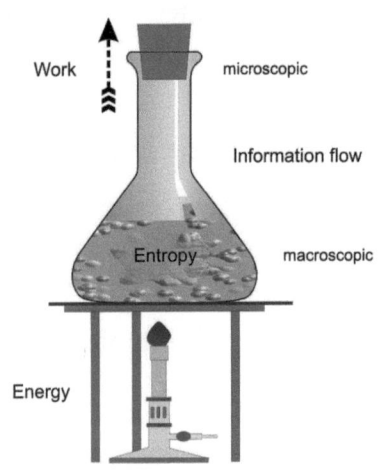

Energy is supplied to a gas-filled piston, which is closed with a stopper, causing it to move outwards. Work is done to overcome friction and due to pressure. What all gas molecules do in detail and how they interact with each other and with the glass walls (=in the microscopic) cannot be determined using mathematical methods. However, it is possible to calculate the work done by the outward movement of the stopper (=in the macroscopic). The energy input increases the entropy (=disorder) of the system. In the non-evaluable microstate, information is generated that can be used to make a statement about the macrostate. At the same time, the environment is informed about the current status of the system.

Fig. 24: Relationship between energy, entropy and information exchange.
Graphic Sedlacek

Entropy changes in any systems may be divided into

☰ Entropy production due to the irreversible processes taking place within a system.

- 目 Entropy flow (=entropy export) across borders into or out of a system.

In the thermodynamic sense, every organism, especially every single cell, is an open system (=dissipative non-equilibrium system) that interacts with its environment. Irreversible processes, i.e., entropy generating processes, are constantly taking place, such as chemical reactions with heat, mass or electrical compensating currents.

A full-grown organism, like every single cell, is in an almost stationary state for long periods of time, apart from regular rhythmic fluctuations. This is only possible with a continued entropy export.

The ongoing irreversible processes play a constructive role in living systems: on the one hand they create order, on the other hand they leave disorder (143). This life-sustaining export of entropy is essentially based on three processes (144):

- 目 heat release
- 目 exchange of matter with the environment
- 目 internal transformation of matter

Accordingly, the release of heat to the environment is a vital process. This is the only way that the devalued energy and thus reduced entropy can be exported. A living organism thus escapes heat death.

According to Shannon (145), information seems to have something to do with probability because it eliminates uncertainty. The more one expects from the message, the more information one receives when fulfilling a certain message, i.e., its "novelty value". The information theory he founded captures statistical information such as the uniqueness of the shape or pattern. Thus, any distinction between two possibilities can be clarified by a single yes-no query. He defined the *bit* as unit information.

"Entropy" was introduced as the measure of the loss of information, for example in data transmissions that create content between thermodynamics and information theory with the following relationship:

Total information of a system =
Random information + Ordered information.

If entropy is viewed as the amount of random information in a system and ordered information is taken as the information of the usable part of the system's energy, then the total information in the system is always greater than or equal to entropy. However, the size of the ordered information in a system is fundamentally much smaller than that of the random information. Therefore, the ordered information can be neglected when viewed roughly and the following applies:

Total information =
Random information = Entropy = Devalued energy.

From this it is to be concluded that the entire information of a system corresponds to the part of the energy that can no longer be used. Regardless of whether the energy is no longer usable or is devalued in relation to the system from which it originates, it remains energy. And the information about the system is equivalent to that. Every real system generates entropy during its work. Entropy, a form of energy that can no longer be used within the system, also generates information that is equivalent to this energy.

If, as in the Boltzmann experiment, the entropy of a macrostate is characterized by the number of possible microstates, then the entropy corresponds to the information that is missing to fully describe the corresponding microstate. Information is then the difference between the entropy of a given macrostate and the entropy of the one with the greatest possible entropy. Entropy thus becomes, as it were, missing information.

5.3.2 Relationship between quantum information and measurement process

The (quantum) information occurring in quantum mechanical systems is normalized with the elementary unit of a quantum bit (*qubit*). In contrast to a classic picture with a yes-no alternative a qubit represents all alternatives at the same time. Mathematical functions can be used to calculate the probability, with which a certain result is expectable in a measurement. Before the "observed" measurement, a qubit is ambiguous and its states are superposed. Its superposition is only canceled by a measurement process. The system is brought into an unambiguous state of physical reality: an abstract qubit becomes a concrete bit.

Based on experimentally verifiable interactions, a physical entity can be derived from a closed system with full applicability of the law of conservation of energy: it consists of a 4-dimensional (metric) reality and at the same time a spaceless and timeless (metric-free) realness (see 5.2 differentiation between reality and realness). Information-processing (=physical measuring process) leads to interactions within the system. The energy is constant in this closed system. Regardless of local appearances and phenomena of realness, as defined above, a metrically inaccessible realness with direct and instantaneous interaction can be conclusively derived. In common it is a real physical entity.

In metric reality, entropy creates an equivalence between statistical-physical information and devalued energy. In the metric-free realness, however, it could be the measurement process that analogously expresses an equivalence between elementary information and inaccessible energy. If, as in the Boltzmann experiment, the entropy of a macrostate is characterized by the number of possible microstates, the measurement process would accurately characterize the information that is missing to describe the corresponding microstate of the metric-free realness.

Could elementary information now be normalized? In his theoretical considerations von Weizsäcker pointed out (146) (147) that all conceivable elementary particles can be built up from binary alternatives, but this would only correspond to a different description of statistical information. Görnitz (148) (149) achieves a normalization using Bekenstein's and Hawking's interventions in the entropy of black holes with the absolute size of the elementary information of elementary particles. In a thought experiment, the entire mass of the universe should be concentrated in a single black hole except for a single H^+-proton still outside. In analogy to the Boltzmann experiment, the entropy of this black hole is to be understood as statistical information that is inaccessibly represented in its interior. When the last H^+-proton enters the black hole, entropy increases. That would correspond exactly to the amount of elementary information that is now being lost to the outer space. This means that a linear relationship can be determined between elementary information and the masses of the black hole and H^+-proton. The elementary information thus corresponds to the mass of the proton.

5.3.3 Interactions in the living via bit and qubit

The last common ancestor LUCA has evolved over time. A single eukaryotic cell gave rise to a cluster of a few cells, which eventually evolved into complex forms containing trillions of cells, culminating in the structure of a human being. In principle, it is possible to supply all of these cells with statistical information about the entropy processes. A single cell typically absorbs "high quality" energy and "devalues" it over time. It is then no longer possible to reverse this process. In order to stay alive itself, i.e., to stay as far away from thermodynamic equilibrium as possible, it exports devalued energy to the environment, mostly in the form of heat. The cell network in the immediate vicinity is thus informed about the condition of the individual cell. The flow of information occurs through changes in the properties of molecules. Their electrons are able to absorb energy as a "networked electron cloud" and thus change their structure. The absorption of, for example, electromagnetic radiation in the form of a real photon ends its existence. In addition to the information associated with the photon, physical energy is also transferred to the absorbing molecule.

The intra and intercellular communication includes, among other things, instructions for protein folding or even the implementation of morphogenetic blueprints. In order to synchronize the many trillions of cells, a controlling information structure must be able to transmit relevant information almost instantaneously across the entire cell network.

According to quantum information theory, timeless and spaceless elementary information condenses into energy or matter through photons, forming the 4-dimensional metric world we know. Electrons, being in a biological quantum field receive information at the moment they oscillatory interact with randomly condensing photons. These can also be entangled and thus become another information carrier: an orbital of a living being belonging to a biological quantum field metrically represents a space in which entangled photons form a quantum channel for the instantaneous transmission of information by quantum teleportation (150) while providing an important classical-physical channel through oscillating molecules and electrons. The information thus transmitted may relate to specific instructions for use stored in a metric-free archive, e.g., protein folding instructions or morpho-genetic blueprints (151).

5.4 Novel measurement techniques as biophysical biomarkers?

The physical concept of information allows statements about conditions of matter or energy, including a biological system. Furthermore, deviations from a "healthy" state could be interpreted as a disease-related disorder and associated with entropy.

According to Boltzmann, the individual behavior of the gas molecules involved in the glass piston experiment cannot be recorded methodically. On the other hand, it is possible to accurately describe the macroscopic behavior of the stopper. With a newly discovered natural constant, the work done becomes calculable and general conclusions can be drawn for the microbehavior of the gas molecules in the piston. Shannon, on the other hand, uses the concept of entropy to characterize the information content of messages. A connection between the concept of information and the entropy of a closed system is established via probabilities.

Findings that Boltzmann gained from the gas-filled glass piston experiment allow trend-setting statements on diagnostics in living systems. Assuming the above case, something else can be observed or measured depending on the perspective. A promising approach for targeted diagnostics would be to record entropy as the information carrier of the system. Deviations from the norm could be perceived as a disturbance and associated with the term "disease." Contrasting the approach of Boltzmann and Shannon with the epistemiological methods of molecular biology, in the following situation arises for a cell:

Molecular biology attempts to describe the microscopic individual behavior and interrelationships of molecules, proteins or enzymes that together lead to a macroscopic understanding of a cell's disease state. This is certainly a promising approach for medical research, but less suitable for non-invasive in vivo diagnostics. If, on the other hand, a biological disorder is understood as a macroscopic (reality) state and the information about its triggering is linked to the statistical entropy of the system, the better method for non-invasive diagnostic procedures in vivo turns out to be. This consists in comparing the entropy of an open system with the measurement of electromagnetic waves as an information vector. Analogously to Boltzmann's considerations, a disorder would be represented macroscopically as a disease that allows conclusions to be drawn about the entropy change of a microsystem, demonstrated here by a cell with all its molecules, proteins or enzymes (152).

5.4.1 Possibilities of an entropy or information-based diagnostics

Understanding a biological disorder as a macroscopic (reality) state and fathoming the information about the triggering of the disturbance via the entropy of the system, seems to be a promising diagnostic approach. Important recent developments in this field have enabled the visualization of tissue microstructure and thus the quantitative mapping of disease-specific endogenous and exogenous substances. With these advances, optical imaging technologies are the upcoming clinical tools for non-invasive and objective diagnosis, therapies initiated and their continuous monitoring. Recent developments include visible and infrared diffuse spectroscopy and imaging, spectral imaging, optical coherence tomography, confocal imaging, molecular imaging and dynamic spectral imaging (73). As an example, the quantification of mitochondrial dynamics in living cells is presented:

For example, a 3D time-lapse imaging method based on photothermal optical coherence microscopy using a novel surface functionalization of gold nanoparticles, is suitable for monitoring mitochondrial dynamics in live HeLa cells. The biocompatible protein-based biopolymer coating contains multiple functional groups that mediate better cellular uptake as well as more efficient mitochondria targeting. The high stability of the gold nanoparticles enables continuous imaging over longer periods of up to 3000 seconds without significant cell damage becoming visible. By combining a temporal auto-correlation analysis with a classical diffusion model, the mitochondrial dynamics can be quantified. Results are presented in 3D maps showing the heterogeneity of diffusion parameters throughout the cell volume (88).

5.4.2 Possibilities of quantum physics based diagnostics

5.4.2.1 Fluorescence resonance energy transfer

Förster-resonance energy transfer or fluorescence resonance energy transfer (FRET) is a physical process of energy transfer. The energy of an excited dye (=donor) is transferred to a second (=acceptor). The energy is transmitted without radiation and not via the emission and absorption of photons (153). Due to the radiation-free energy transfer, it is not directly detectable. However, the consequences, namely the decrease in the radiation intensity and the fluorescence lifetime of the donor dye and the acceptor dyes responsible for the radiation emission, can be detected by the acceptor emission. The fluorescence microscope or the fluorimeter, for example, are suitable for these detections.

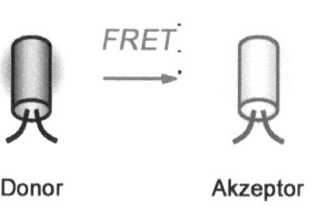

Fig. 25: Distance-dependent energy transfer from an excited donor to an acceptor via the Förster mechanism.

An entanglement state is clearly represented with FRET (Fig. 25). According to this, an oscillation is induced in the acceptor by the excited donor, which preserves and maintains the quantum mechanical properties of the spins of the donor and acceptor dye. The energy transferred to the acceptor dye can also be emitted again in the form of radiation. On the other hand, the energy transferred is no longer available to the donor dye for a direct radiation emission.

For example, the light-harvesting complex in photosynthetic organisms is based on FRET. In molecular biology, Förster resonance energy transfer is often used in DNA-based methods. Here, for example, dye-coupled DNA oligonucleotides are deployed, in which an energy transfer is observed by duplex formation or alternatively terminated by destruction of their tertiary structure. This is used, among other things, as an analytical tool in polymerase chain reaction (PCR), mutation analysis and determining the concentration of DNA and RNA.

5.4.2.2 Electron transport through porphyrins

Porphyrins are organic molecules in the central region of macromolecules, such as chlorophyll and hemoglobin, with a metal atom in their center that determines their specific function. The importance of these molecules in the field of molecular electronics lies in their ease of transferring electrons from one region to another (154) (Fig.26).

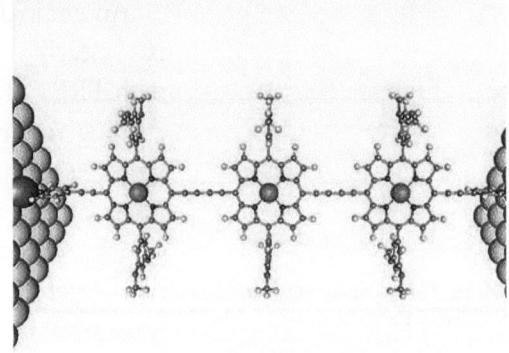

Fig. 26: Gold surfaces connected by three units of porphyrin.
By Centro de Investigación en Nanomateriales y Nanotecnología. Usage Restrictions None.

Electron transport is synonymous with energy transport or electric current flow. The ease of electron transport in porphyrins resembles a quantum mechanical tunneling effect: electrons have a predictable probability of disappearing from one location and instead reappearing at a different location outside of the original molecule. Such effects are associated on the one hand with somehow acquired energy. That is because it takes more energy to traverse space than is available. On the other hand, the spatial and temporal dimensions of classical physics are abolished. Tunneling is instantaneous with no intermediate state, meaning faster than the speed of light. For example, if a tunneled electron reappears at a different location, it will have the same quantum properties as before tunneling. And if the electron was entangled with other electrons before tunneling, this is also the case afterwards (155).

As with the light-harvesting complexes in plants, quantum mechanical entanglement also exists in porphyrins. As a universal principle, low-energy photons are collected until the start of the biochemical process. These interact with the electron participating in the biochemical process and give it their energy. The electron is

88

instantaneously tunneled from the interaction site to that of the biochemical process.

5.4.2.3 Principal possibility of detecting quantum effects in hemoglobin

Quantum biological interactions in living structures can be clearly demonstrated from the previous illustration: oxygen O_2, inhaled through respiration, is required for the oxyhydrogen reaction to generate energy in the mitochondrial respiratory chain. Hemoglobin porphyrins supply the energy required to bind O_2 or CO_2 in a process explainable by FRET.

5.4.3 Are diagnostically and therapeutically integrated procedures possible in principle?

In order to be able to detect objects without significant interactions, an interaction-free measurement (IFM) is required to avoid any damage that may occur. Based on quantum channel theory, a Mach-Zehnder-like interferometer could use a Quantum-Zeno-effect as a quantum-based analysis technique (156) (157). From an integrative perspective, such a "diagnostic" approach should be followed by a "therapeutic" one at the same time.

As an illustrative example, the division process of a cell during mitosis is chosen. It is likely that normal mirror-like mitosis is organized by quantum coherence between microtubule-based centrioles and the mitotic spindles. This ensures exact complementary duplication of the genome of daughter cells as well as recognition of their respective cell boundaries. Thus, a quantum state of cyto- or nuclear plasma is generated in combination with quantum-optical properties of centrioles at physiological temperature.

With low-energy laser illumination in the range of 635 or 830 nm, increased cell division can be triggered immediately in a cell culture with a laser. Apparently the centriolar replication and thus the consecutive cell division is stimulated. If centrioles now react sensitively to coherent light with an increased replication rate, they could conversely be selectively disturbed by a higher intensity during mitosis, e.g., above a certain temperature threshold that could be used as a therapeutic option, e.g., in cancer treatment (158).

However, laser illumination can also be used more elegantly: when entangled centrioles interact with condensed photons, therapeutic options arise due to the advantageous properties of radiation-generated centrosomes or centrioles. Under defined conditions, such as when a certain organism or tissue is selected, normal centrioles should exhibit specific quantum-optical properties that would need to be verified by some sort of selection technique.

From these perspectives, it would be possible to examine normal healthy cells of an affected patient, such as one with cancer, to identify the normal cell-specific properties of the centrioles. In principle, the identical and coherent photons generated with these properties could also be used destructively against malignant cells. However, not under the same conditions just described since relatively low laser energy is used in this mode. Rather, an attempt should then be made to reprogram or stimulate a redifferentiation of centrioles with the aim of converting tumor cells into a healthy and differentiated tissue (158) (159) (160).

5.5 How might human life function from a quantum biological point of view?

Based on the genome of archaea and proteobacteria, a biophysical information system has evolved from which living humans have emerged with superconscious, subconscious and perceived subjectivity. As a self-organizing dissipative non-equilibrium system in a biological space-time construct, it constantly attempts to escape from thermodynamic equilibrium through sophisticated energy management and thus maintain its existence by avoiding death from heat or cold.

In quantum physics, isothermally living organisms can be imagined as structures similar to liquid crystals. Quantum associated processes, such as coherences in biological systems as prolonged electromagnetic correlation between physically separated oscillating-electric dipoles, explain how superconducting properties occur between molecules or dipole clusters under isothermal conditions in different cellular or anatomical structures. Among other things, nucleotides in a single DNA strand can be modeled as a coupled chain of harmonic quantum oscillators with dipole-dipole interactions between nearest molecular neighbors. Subatomic structures are able to overcome a potential barrier through tunneling effects without the necessary energy being available at that moment.

5.5.1 Pure and everyday coincidence

In addition to a pure, objective, uncontrollable random element, there is another fundamentally deterministic one with non-objective properties. The latter as a more everyday coincidence is modeled by environmental influences, genetic predisposition and individual behavior. Entangled photons, on the other hand, which, for example, refer to a metric-free morphogenetic blueprint, condense purely by chance according to quantum mechanical laws. Through information-processing, elementary information from the metric-free realness gets into the 4-dimensional reality and thus receives its real-physical existence.

5.5.2   Evolutive Awareness (see definition 5.1)

Adaptive mutation is a mechanism by which organisms increase mutation rates in response to rising selection pressures. There is evidence that mutations can be manipulated at will (161). In quantum physics, such phenomena of awareness are comparable to the Inverse quantum zeno effect: a series of measurements at short intervals on the quantum system forces it to evolve in a certain direction. At the same time, coupling to the environment allows a cell to probe possible and useful mutational spectra during a coherent state. While cellular mechanisms may act on "possibilities" in how a measuring device works, they cannot create facts because quantum measurement requires a self-referential awareness operation. However, if a meaningful mutation pattern is aware recognized, the phenotypic expression has a favorable effect on the organism due to the available genetic information, coherence occurs and the genetic mutation becomes factual in a specific configuration (162).

A mutation caused by the displacement of a single hydrogen atom from its originally neighboring atom may itself be viewed as a quantum mechanical tunneling process. If necessary, information-processing and self-organization are set in motion, with the help of which the selection is consciously controlled at an elementary level. To a certain extent, nature voluntarily decides for itself how it evolves. Evolution in this context has a kind of symbiotic relationship between aware self-organization and objective chance.

5.5.3 Integrity of the biological space-time construction

The integrity as physical unit of an organism and the trouble-free course of all biological processes is guaranteed by physical rules of the 4-dimensional world and immanently modeled by biological quantum processes.

Structure

The mass of electrons, unlike living structures, seems to exist indefinitely. Molecules or associations are formed by chemical bonds. The atoms involved in biological molecules are bound together by well-known types of bonds and interactions. These include covalent, ionic and hydrogen bonding, hydrophobic interactions and van der Waals forces. Covalent bonds form very stable structures, while weak hydrogen bonds, which are common in biomolecules, play an important role in biological processes such as protein folding or other structural formation. While animate structures can release devalued energy into the environment and thus preserve their integrity, inanimate ones have reached an irreversible state of thermodynamic equilibrium, colloquially meaning "death".

Shape and form

Information about morphogenetic blueprints of biological structures is found neither in DNA nor in other biomolecules. Presumably, such blueprints are stored metric-free in the biological quantum fields of the associated living system. Entangled photons condensing as a result of fluctuation and subsequently interacting with electrons of an orbital in living structures would retrieve information from the corresponding memory for morphogenetic blueprints: as real-physical information carriers, such photons are then able to transmit morphogenetic information to trillions of cells.

Aging

Environmental influences, genetic factors, individual lifestyle or cell death due to acute disorders modulate the normal aging process. The cell regenerates itself by regulatory processes, adapts its performance, become senescent or dies through programmed cell death. Over time, the regulatory ability to compensate becomes exhausted and efficiency decreases. From a quantum physics point of view and based on biological quantum fields, aging is thought to be mediated through a deformation of space-time geometry, leading to a change in cell architecture.

5.5.4   Life between health and disease

Every single cell requires high-quality energy to stay alive. The utilization of this energy accelerates the disorder within the cell, which without countermeasures would reach a maximum and then lead to heat death.

Order

Order is created by entropy export as heat release to the environment. Two functions are fulfilled at the same time: passing on information to the environment and maintaining a physiological milieu for optimal living conditions. Heat, on the other hand, is necessary for the activities of functional proteins and protection by the immune system. Excessive cooling leads to the cessation of life-support processes and ultimately death from the cold. Under normal physiological conditions, life-sustaining processes run regularly. The environment absorbs heat and thus receives information about the "health" of a cell. Thermodynamically, life is an attempt to exist between heat and cold death.

Disease

Purely by chance, the electromagnetic waves associated with information-processing condense as photons that create space and time. The photons that become real in a biological quantum field also contribute to an entropy change of the corresponding living system. When disorder accelerates, it signals a disruption that manifests itself at the macroscopic (reality) level as a deviation from normal health. Finally, decoherent states that occur in a liquid-crystal-like biological structure also deforms the space-time geometry of the associated quantum field, which subsequently leads to aging and alteration in the architecture of a cell. If subatomic structures have overcome a potential barrier through tunneling effects, permanent mutations in the genome may also come about. Over time, normal DNA function becomes progressively compromised, resulting in more or less severe genomic and proteomic instability that ultimately manifests as disease.

The development process of such a disease is modulated by mutations that arose purely by chance or as deterministic coincidence as a result of environmental influences, genetic and epigenetic factors or individual lifestyle. Mediated by tunnel effects or otherwise, mutations result in modified cells with altered morphogenetic properties. Modified cells also affect intra- and intercellular communication channels. The comparison of normal and modified cells is initially possible in a multicellular system. If the counter-regulation fails, biological control circuits break down until finally the life-sustaining system fails (163).

6 The mitochondrial energy aspect from a quantum biological perspective: The quantum mitochondrion.

Quantum mechanical oscillations occur in almost all biological systems. With the discovery of the mitochondrial oscillators, an interaction between the generation of free reactive oxygen species (ROS) and the electron transport chain (ETC) could be described (164). The chemiosmotic coupling during photosynthesis and the fractionated oxyhydrogen reaction in the respiratory chain, is an ETC-mediated process that efficiently ensures the production or utilization of glucose, for example. The high efficiency is due to quantum effects, some of which have now become well-known in mitochondria, such as the tunnel effect: In biological systems, electrons not only move themselves along covalent bonds within a molecule, but can also easily jump distances in the nanometer range. Tunneling is the ability of electrons, protons or photons to cross an otherwise insurmountable potential barrier at the sub-atomic level (165) (166).

6.1 Electron transport chain

In the mitochondrial inner membrane, electron transfers are mediated by electron tunneling during random collisions: Ubiquinone and Cytochrome C transfer electrons between key enzyme complexes in the respiratory chain. Both electron carriers diffuse rapidly along the inner membrane of the mitochondria. The expected rate of random collisions between these mobile carriers and the slower diffusing enzyme complexes roughly match the observed rate of electron transfer. Each complex accepts and donates an electron in milliseconds (165).

The orderly transfer of electrons along the respiratory chain, can be fully attributed to the peculiarities of the functional interaction between the components of the chain: each of the electron carriers interacts only with its sequential neighbors and without short-circuiting. This quantum mechanical property turns out to be crucial for an orderly progression of the process. The separation between the carriers prevents short circuits that would occur when a carrier with a low redox potential collides with a carrier with a high one. Protection is assured when an electron is embedded deep enough in a protein and prevented from tunneling to an unsuitable partner (167).

6.2 Enzymes

As early as 1941, a behavior of electrons that deviated from standard thermodynamics was observed in enzymatic reactions (168) (169) and later identified as quantum tunneling. Such effects are not only limited to electrons, but are also found with protons (170).

Alcohol dehydrogenase (ADH) experiments provided the first direct evidence for proton tunneling in enzyme reactions. It is a yeast enzyme tasked with transferring a proton from one alcohol molecule to another molecule (NAD+), creating NADH (=nicotinamide adenine dinucleotide hydride). The detection is based on the method of the kinetic isotope effect (171). Tunneling effects are also influenced by the mass of the subatomic structures involved. Small particles like electrons are easier to tunnel, but heavy ones present more problems unless they have to travel only a very short distance. This is why a proton can tunnel in enzyme reactions even though it has a mass 2000 times higher than an electron. It involves moving a hydrogen atom from one place to another, for example to break the bond in a protein chain. These effects are largely temperature dependent. While some of the quantum properties of inorganic substances are best demonstrated at a temperature close to absolute zero, life functions especially in the normothermic regime and also under isothermal conditions.

The enzyme molecule holds substrates such as a protein chain and a single hydrogen molecule in place during its process. With its functional part, the active center of the enzyme, for example, the dissolution of peptide bonds is accelerated catalytically: the enzyme keeps the peptide bond in the unstable transition state. This must be set before the binding can be broken. The substrates are fixed in exactly the right positions by weak chemical bonds, so that bonds in the protein chain can be dissolved in a targeted manner. Essentially, the forces are mediated by electrons shared between the substrate and the enzyme. This carefully studied process at the molecular control center is fundamentally different from the thermodynamically mediated chaotic molecular motion in a cell. In the interaction of highly structured biomolecules in organized tissues and in all cells, enzymes actively stimulate change processes that affect the entire organism (172).

6.3   Mitochondrial dynamics (fusion and fission)

Mild stress or a reduced food intake favor the process of mitochondrial fusion and increase oxidative phosphorylation. Fission fragmentation, on the other hand, is induced by severe stress, excess nutrients, disease or inflammation, usually resulting in mitophagy and reduces oxidative phosphorylation (86).

The mitochondrial dynamics with fusion and fission processes modulate field strengths at the cellular level. In vitro experiments with fused mitochondria have demonstrated electric fields resembling those in electrical conductors (173) (174). This is relevant because chemical and biochemical processes rely on electromagnetic interactions. Electrostatic force fields provide the ability to release kinetic energy that affects cell function and shape. Static electric or magnetic force fields can be described quantum mechanically, which would correspond to the principle of energy transfer with vibrational coupling between mitochondria and microtubules (175). According to principles of quantum physics, control over morphology and function derives from mitochondrial dynamics (176).

6.4   DNA mutation

The stable transmission of genetic information is ensured by the canonical structure of DNA. When the proton required for hydrogen bonding between complementary base pairs changes position within a nucleic acid despite transfer barriers, a newly formed tautomer prevents binding at the original site but allows binding at a different one. Each point mutation that occurs in this way interferes with the trouble-free transmission of genetic information (177) (178).

Quantum effects exist in biochemical processes such as protein synthesis in DNA macromolecules. As a prerequisite for a quantum entangled system, corresponding elements must interact. This becomes possible, when they tend to stay in a defined environment. An electron cloud created by the helical shape of DNA provides ideal conditions for such interactions (Fig.27).

The high efficiency in selecting nucleotides during DNA replication is due to quantum effects in the involved protons acting between nucleotides and DNA polymerase (179). Similar to superconductivity at a temperature close to absolute zero, coherence in a DNA electron cloud occurs over longer distances, even under isothermal conditions and temperatures around 37° Celsius (180). In terms of quantum physics, this scenario can be understood as an entanglement of direct neighbors in the electron cloud of the DNA strand. A coupled chain is modeled as harmonic oscillators

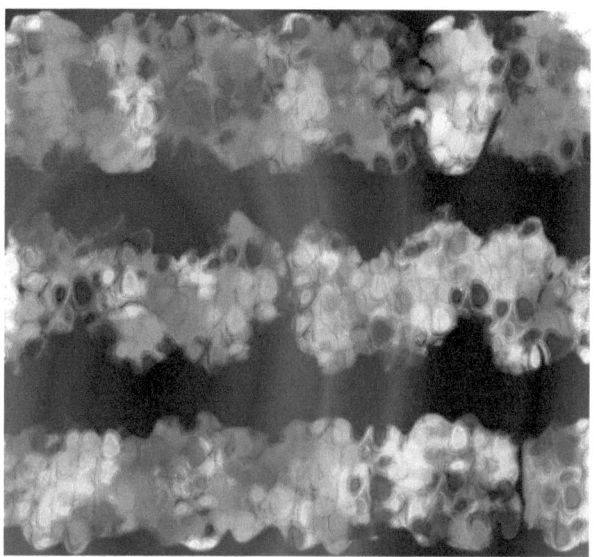

Fig. 27: Visualisation DNA electron cloud
Grafic: Sedlacek

with dipole-dipole interactions between direct neighbors bound by van der Waals forces (181) (182).

DNA repair processes are also subject to such effects. For example, when a bulge is formed by dimerization of adjacent pyrimidines by ultraviolet irradiation, flavoprotein photolyase is able to repair the deformed DNA. It cleaves the covalently linked pyrimidines via electron transfer, allowing them to return to their normal monomeric form. Light of a certain wavelength is required for this process. One of the photolyase cofactors is an antenna molecule that absorbs light at longer wavelength (blue) (183).

Quantum entanglement in antenna molecules serves to collect, add and forward lower energy photons to an electron that requires a discretely higher amount of energy to rise to a higher energy level. If individual photons hit an electron with too little energy, there is no interaction. A higher energy level could then not be reached. Therefore, the energy of the photon that is to interact

101

with an electron must be sufficiently large. However, not all light photons have enough energy to excite the electrons of the invest-igated protein molecules so strongly that an interaction occurs. If, on the other hand, the electrons of several protein molecules are entangled, they behave as a single system. The energy from multiple incident low-energy photons is then treated as if it came from a single photon of higher energy. An electron within the entangled system then absorbs as much energy as it needs to rise to a higher energy level. Because only discrete amounts of energy are absorbed, some of it may remain. This excess energy is either used to increase the kinetic energy of the electron, or a photon is emitted whose energy amount exactly corresponds to the excess energy (184).

6.5 Reactive oxygen species (ROS)

As an example of a quantum biologically mediated cell regulation, reactive oxygen species (ROS) are used in living cells, which are influenced by coherent electron spin dynamics. ROS partitioning appears to be mediated through the formation of spin-correlated radical pairs upon activation of molecular oxygen O_2 by reduced flavoenzymes. Oscillating magnetic fields at the Zeeman resonance alter the relative yields of ROS products from cellular superoxide O_2^- and hydrogen peroxide H_2O_2, indicating a coherent singlet-triplet mixing at the point of ROS formation. Furthermore, the orientation dependence of magnetic stimulation leading to specific changes in ROS levels increases either mitochondrial respiration or glycolysis. Such results demonstrate quantum effects in live cell cultures bridging atomic and cellular levels by linking ROS partitioning to cellular bioenergetics (185).

6.6 Protein folding

Protein electron transfer mechanisms exist at the molecular and cellular level. They vary from coherent tunneling over long distances to thermally activated jumps. In order to understand such processes, the mechanisms at the molecular level must be fundamentally known. Accordingly, electron transfer (ET) in proteins plays a central role in many biological functions, particularly in bioenergetic processes. All ET types exhibit a quantum mechanical nature. Accordingly, not only protein folding but also protein function, in particular the electron-mediated energy transfer, is subject to quantum-associated mechanisms (186).

As a result of a central dogma of molecular biology, the protein structure with the amino acid sequence of the fold and cofactors

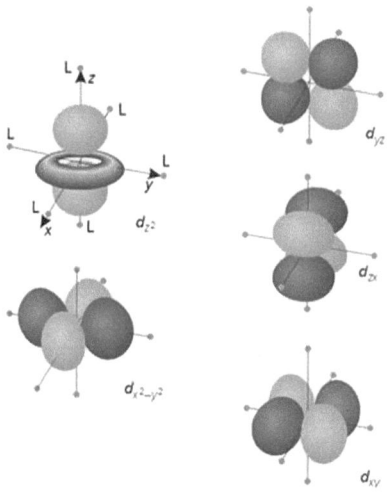

Fig. 28: Simplified forms of the different d-orbitals. An isosurface of the probability density is shown for the respective orbitals.
By J3D3 - Own work, GFDL, https://commons.wikimedia.org/w/index.php?curid=3525412

determine the function of the protein. The dome-model of the probability of electrons, this time to describe the electron orbitals along the amino acid strand of folded proteins, cannot pinpoint the exact position of an electron in an atom at any given time (Fig.28).

However, the space in an atom in which the electron resides can be described with a certain degree of probability: the space in which the electron resides at least 90% of the time is commonly referred to as the orbital. Molecules there have orbital overlap, with the electron wave functions either adding or subtracting depending on whether the molecular orbitals are bonding or antibonding.

For a protein with so many atoms, the orbital space is very large compared to the nanoscale: If you were to assign a proton the size of a soccer ball, the associated electron could occupy a position up to 10 kilometers away. Within this orbital space there are also those electrons capable of interacting with purely randomly condensed photons. It is conceivable that protein folding and the orbital space altered by folding is not an accidental result of the evolution of proteins, but is somehow related to the function of the protein. Then the electron orbital volume of a protein would have evolved along functional lines. On average, sufficient activation energy is collected and reserved for its specific function. Antenna molecules in the context of photosynthesis are an example of a highly efficient "collecting" of photons. Taken together, there is clearly a universal principle according to which the functionality of a protein is determined by its folding. Quantum connected it is an information driven evolutionary process.

6.7 Do aware processes check protein quality control?

The reason for the defective protein folding is complex. It is mainly gene mutations that lead to changes in the amino acid se-

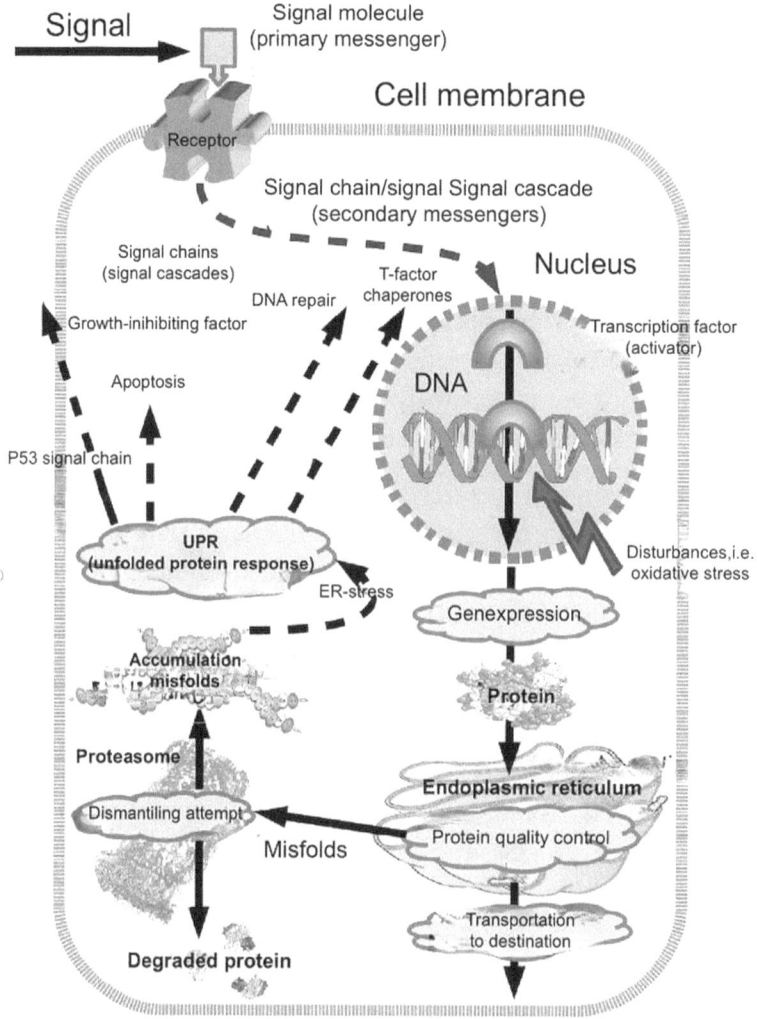

Fig. 29: Schematic summary of the major regulatory processes associated with gene expression in a eukaryotic cell.
Graphic Sedlacek

quence. In addition, toxic stress or exposure to radiation also conduct to erroneous changes in DNA over the course of life. The amino acid sequences formed by the biosynthesis of proteins have a direct impact on secondary and tertiary structure or on the protein folding process. Errors in transcription or translation or through the incorporation of toxins during protein synthesis may also lead to misfolding. The question therefore arises as to which biophysical models are useable to meaningfully describe what happens in connection with protein quality control (Fig. 29).

The effect of toxins on DNA or proteins may be described in classical physical terms, but not that of radiation or mutation. The latter is also a matter of events at the subatomic level. So when gene mutations are triggered by radiation or proton tunneling, a quantum biological discussion makes sense.

Whether a protein is correctly folded is determined at the quality center by proofreading at the subatomic level. This process determines whether the protein is fully folded or not. There are more than 20,000 different primary proteins in the human body. Up to several hundred protein species can be synthesized by mRNA splicing and subsequent modification of the primary protein by enzymes, in humans up to 1,000,000. In protein quality control, how time critical is it to ensure that each of these protein types is correctly folded? To calculate a single millisecond of a protein folding process, the supercomputer Anton needs up to 100 days of computing time (187). On the other hand, if the chaperones involved in this task know in milliseconds whether a protein is completely or correctly folded, then a huge database must be running in the background that is accessed, or there is some kind of biological quantum computer that can do the tasks faster. Regardless of explanations based on classical physical aspects, information-processing at the quantum level seems most plausible: chaperones probably act aware.

6.8   Meaning of pure chance

In humans, some tissue types are millions of times more susceptible to cancer than others. Apparently, the lifetime cancer risk of many different species is strongly correlated with the total number of normal self-renewing cell divisions for tissue homeostasis. There is evidence that only a third of the variation in tissue cancer risk is attributable to environmental factors or hereditary predisposition. The majority is due to the randomness of mutations in DNA-replication of normal, non-cancerous stem cells (188).

In principle, coincidences can be distinguished. The directed, non-objective and fundamentally deterministic coincidence that we are familiar with is modeled by everyday environmental influences and predisposition. Pure chance, on the other hand, is objective and non-deterministic according to quantum theory and is also referred to as quantum chance. The latter is attributed to the principle of fluctuation with subsequent condensation of photons, the emergence of "something" from "nothing", without regularity, i.e., purely by chance.

In the scenario presented, cancer arises from a combination of pure chance and deterministic coincidence involving environmental factors and predisposition. Whether an exposed person develops cancer or not is largely a matter of luck (189).

7 Summary and outlook

The (patho-)physiological mechanism presented, which particularly emphasizes the development process of a sporadic form of Alzheimer's disease at the cellular level, can in principle also be transferred to other cells with high energy consumption such as the heart or skeletal muscles. This may result in new therapeutic options in the treatment of heart failure or sarcopenia. A transfer of findings from the investigation of homoplasmic mitochondrial diseases to heteroplasmic ones is also conceivable.

In summary, the onset of the sporadic form of Alzheimer's disease is primarily due to a normal aging process, followed by a combination of pure chance and deterministic coincidence involving environmental factors and predisposition. Whether an exposed person falls ill or not is largely a question of fate.

Remarkably, the reduction to a molecular biological or genetic origin has not made a satisfactory contribution to the understanding of the development of this disease. Only from an emergent perspective including energetic and genetic aspects, has the view of its pathoetiogenesis become clearer. At the same time, an exceedingly complex background is pointed out. And here the energetic factor clearly stands out. The high efficiency of biological energy utilization and ATP energy production allows conclusions to be drawn about physical processes, which will be no longer be explained solely on the basis of classical physics. Different properties and processes of life can clearly be traced back to quantum biological principles, albeit in a non-trivial way:

This is how our common ancestor, the Last Universal Common Ancestor (LUCA) evolved over time. From a single eukaryotic cell, a small-cell assemblage first developed, from which complex forms with trillions of cells finally emerged, culminating in the structure of a human being. The entire ontogenetic or phylogenetic development process is stored as statistical information in the DNA. In principle, it is possible to supply all of these cells with statistical information solely by means of the entropy process. However, this form of communication has proven to be completely inadequate, for example for protein folding instructions or the implementation of morphogenetic blueprints. In order to synchronize the many trillions of cells, the information structure control must be able to convey relevant information without delay across the entire cell network.

It is now clear that such a complex flow of information can be realized with the help of quantum biology. The electrons of a corresponding orbital in a biological quantum field receive information by oscillating with randomly condensing photons. In metric reality, these become physical information carriers and are thus able to synchronize the development steps of trillions of cells. The condensed photons originating from the metric-free realness can also be part of an entangled system and thus become another information carrier: An orbital belonging to a biological quantum field will be both the space in which entangled photons transfer information via a quantum channel faster than the speed of light by quantum teleportation and via an important classical physical channel through oscillating molecules and electrons. The information thus transmitted may also relate to specific instructions for use, instructions for protein folding and morphogenetic blueprints, stored in a metric-free information repository.

According to recent findings, animal and plant life originally arose due to quantum mechanical effects such as tunneling or coherence (190), while competition and stress were constant drivers of natural selection. In this context, adaptive mutation is a selection-driving mechanism for organisms to correspondingly increase mutation rates under developmental pressure (191). Information-processing and self-organization processes that are set in motion are aware controlled on an elementary level. On this path, nature decides to a certain extent deliberately for itself how it evolves. From this point of view, evolution stands in a symbiotic relationship between conscious self-organization and objective chance as well as everyday coincidence.

At the end of this exciting journey, the question of an original life principle arises: what actually makes living beings alive?

Life and development processes follow a non-linear dynamic and strive for disordered states. Only then do tendencies towards heterogeneity, diversification, differentiation and instability develop. Living beings embody systems with very high potential energies and at the same time represent a high degree of order maintained by self-organization against all disturbing tendencies. The living differs from the inanimate primarily through its sophisticated energy management. It escapes thermodynamic equilibrium and maintains its existence by avoiding heat or cold death.

There is one another factor that is probably the deciding one: As far as we know today, in an evolutionary process through information-processing that requires some form of awareness, life was enabled to interact directly and instantaneously in nonlocal metric-free realness *and* in 4-dimensional metric reality at the subatomic level.

8 Bibliography

Another view of the development of the sporadic form of Alzheimer's disease

Neuronal mitochondrial energetics / Introduction

1) Alzheimer's disease: the amyloid cascade hypothesis. Hardy JA, Higgins GA. Science.1992; 256(5054):184-5.

2) The Alzheimer's Disease Mitochondrial Cascade Hypothesis. Swerdlow RH, Burns JM, Khan SH. J Alzheimers Dis. 2010; 20(Suppl 2): 265-279. doi: 10.3233/JAD-2010-100339

What is currently known about Alzheimer's disease?

Amyloid Cascade

3) Markers of apoptosis and models of programmed cell death in Alzheimer's disease. Hugon J, Terro F, Esclaire F. J Neural Transm-Supp.2000; 59(59): 125-31. doi: 10.1007/978-3-7091-6781-6_15

4) The Inflammatory Form of Cerebral Amyloid Angiopathy or "Cerebral Amyloid Angiopathy-Related Inflammation" (CAARI). Kirshner HS, Bradshaw M. Curr Neurol Neurosci Rep. 2015; 15(8): 54. doi: 10.1007/s11910-015-0572-y

5) Intracellular amyloid-beta in Alzheimer's disease. LaFerla FM, Green KN, Oddo S. Nat Rev Neurosci. 2007; 8(7): 499-509. doi: 10.1038/nrn2168

6) Simulated cytoskeletal collapse via tau degradation. Sendek A, Fuller HR, Hayre NR et al. PLoS One. 2014; 9(8): e104965. doi: 10.1371/journal.pone.0104965

7) Noncognitive symptoms of early Alzheimer disease. A longitudinal analysis. Masters MC, Morris JC, Roe CM. Neurology. 2015; 84(6): 617-622. doi: 10.1212/WNL.0000000000001238

8) Non-cognitive symptoms in early- and late-onset dementia. Sadanand S, Shivakumar P,Bharath S et al. Alzheimer's & Dementia.2015; 7(11) Supplement: 243-244. doi: https://doi.org/10.1016/j.jalz.2015.07.297

Diagnostic possibilities

9) TREM2 variants: new keys to decipher Alzheimer disease pathogenesis. Colonna M, Wang Y. Nat Rev Neurosci. 2016; 17: 201-207. doi: 10.1038/nrn.2016.7.

Therapeutic options

10) Conserved epigenomic signals in mice and humans reveal immune basis of Alzheimer's disease. Gjoneska E, Pfenning AR, Mathys H. Nature. 2015; 518(7539): 365-9. doi: 10.1038/nature14252

11) Alzheimer's disease drug development pipeline: 2017. Cummings J, Lee G, Mortsdorf T et al. Alzheimer's & Dementia. Translational Research & Clinical Interventions 2017; 3 (3): 367-384.
doi: https://doi.org/10.1016/j.trci.2017.05.002

Mitochondrial aspects

12) Mitochondrial abnormalities in Alzheimer brain: mechanistic implications. Bubber P, Haroutunian V, Fisch G et al. Ann Neurol. 2005; 57(5): 695-703. doi: 10.1002/ana.20474

13) Impaired Platelet Mitochondrial Activity in Alzheimer's Disease and Mild Cognitive Impairment. Valla J, Schneider L, Niedzielko T. Mitochondrion. 2006; 6(6): 323-330. doi: https://doi.org/10.1016/j.mito.2006.10.004

14) Mutations in mitochondrial-encoded cytochrome c oxidase subunits I, II and III genes detected in Alzheimer's disease using single-strand conformation polymorphism. Hamblet NS, Ragland B, Ali M et al. Electrophoresis. 2006; 27(2): 398-408. doi: 10.1002/elps.200500420

15) Amyloid-β peptide induces mitochondrial dysfunction by inhibition of preprotein maturation. Mossmann D, Vögtle FN, Taskin AA et al. Cell Metab. 2014; 20(4): 662-9. doi: 10.1016/j.cmet.2014.07.024

16) Progressive increase in mtDNA 3243A>G heteroplasmy causes abrupt transcriptional reprogramming. Picard M, Zhang J, Hancock S, et al. Proc Natl Acad Sci. 2014; 111(38): E4033-42. doi: 10.1073/pnas.1414028111

Side view: Quality control during protein folding

17) Identifying and validating biomarkers for Alzheimer's disease. Humpel C. Trends Biotechnol. 2011; 29(1): 26-32. doi: 10.1016/j.tibtech.2010.09.007

18) Potential for primary prevention of Alzheimer's disease: an analysis of population-based data. Norton S, Matthews FE, Barnes DE et al. Lancet Neurology. 2016; 13: 788-794, doi: 10.1016/S1474-4422(14)70136-X

19) Members of the Hsp70 Family recognize distinct Types of Sequences to execute ER Quality Control. Behnke J, Mann MJ, Scruggs FL et al. Mol Cell. 2016; 63(5): 739-52. doi: 10.1016/j.molcel.2016.07.012

Characteristics of cellular mitochondria

20) Endosymbiotic theories for eukaryote origin. Martin WF, Garg S, Zimorski V. Philos Trans R Soc Lond B Biol Sci. 2015; 370(1678): 20140330. doi: 10.1098/rstb.2014.0330

21) Bioenergetic role of mitochondrial fusion and fission. Westermann B. Biochim Biophys Acta. 2012; 10(1817): 1833-1838. doi: 10.1016/j.bbabio.2012.02.033

Energy production: Respiratory chain

Side view: Electron transport chain (ETC) / Side view: Special features of the porphyrins and enzymes / Mutation: effect on mitochondrial DNA

22) Sequence analysis of cDNAs for the human and bovine ATP synthase b-subunit: Mitochondrial DNA genes sustain seventeen times more mutations. Wallace DC, Ye JH, Neckelmann SN et al. Curr Genet. 1987; 12: 81-90.

23) MITOMAP A human mitochondrial genome database. (www.mitomap.org)

24) Mitochondrial DNA genetics and the heteroplasmy conundrum in evolution and disease. Wallace DC, Chalkia D. Cold Spring Harb Perspect Biol. 2013; 5(11): a021220. doi: 10.1101/cshperspect.a021220

Side view: Mutation, Methylation

25) Molecular enzymology of mammalian DNA methyltransferases. Jeltsch A. Curr Top Microbiol Immunol. 2006; 301: 203-25.

Damage: Oxidative stress, Reactive oxygen species, Aging

Reactive oxygen species

26) In vivo ROS production and use of oxidative stress-derived biomarkers to detect the onset of diseases such as Alzheimer's disease, Parkinson's disease and diabetes. Umeno A, Biju V, Yoshida Y. Free Radic Res. 2017; 51(4): 413-427. doi:10.1080/10715762.2017.1315114.

27) Oxidative Stress, Synaptic Dysfunction and Alzheimer's Disease. Tönnies E, Trushina E. J Alzheimers Dis. 2017; 57(4): 1105-1121. doi: 10.3233/JAD-161088

Aging

28) Molecular medical basis of age-specific diseases. Ganten D, Ruckpaul K. Springer-Verlag Berlin Heidelberg. 2004. ISBN 978-3-642-18741-4.

29) Mitochondrial DNA mutations in neurodegeneration. Keogh MJ, Chinnery PF. Biochim Biophys Acta. 2015; 11(1847): 1401-1411. doi: 10.1016/j.bbabio.2015.05.015

30) Mitochondrial dysfunction and oxidative stress in neurodegenerative diseases. Lin MT, Beal MF. Nature. 2006;443(7113):787-95. doi: 10.1038/nature05292

31) Mitochondrial DNA variation in human evolution, degenerative disease and aging. Wallace DC. Am J Hum Genet. 1995 Aug; 57(2): 201-223.

Regulation: Mitochondrial dynamics (fusion, fission)

32) Mitochondrial Dynamics - Mitochondrial Fission and Fusion in Human Diseases. Stephen L, Archer SL. N Engl J Med. 2013; 369: 2236-2251. doi: 10.1056/NEJMra1215233

33) Disturbed mitochondrial dynamics and neurodegenerative disorders. Burté F, Carelli V, Chinnery PF et al. Nat Rev Neurol. 2015 1:11-24. doi: 10.1038/nrneurol.2014.228

34) Diet impact on mitochondrial bioenergetics and dynamics. Putti R, Raffaella Sica R, Migliaccio V et al. Front Physiol. 2015; 6: 109. doi: 10.3389/fphys.2015.00109

35) Structural Heterogeneity of the Mitochondria Induced by the Microtubule Cytoskleleton. Sukhorukov VM, Michael Meyer-Hermann M. Scientific Reports. 2015 Sep 11. 5:13924. doi: 10.1038/srep13924.

36) Mitochondrial dynamics and neurodegeneration. Bingwei L. Curr Neurol Neurosci Rep. 2009; 3: 212-219.

37) Impairing the Mitochondrial Fission and Fusion Balance: A New Mechanism of Neurodegeneration. Andrew B, Knott AB, Bossy-Wetzel E. Ann N Y Acad Sci. 2008; 1147: 283-292. doi: 10.1196/annals.1427.030

38) Defects in Mitochondrial Dynamics and Metabolomic Signatures of Evolving Energetic Stress in Mouse Models of Familial Alzheimer's Disease. Trushina E, Nemutlu E, Zhang S et al. PLoS One. 2012; 7(2): e32737. doi: 10.1371/journal.pone.0032737

Signaling: Senescence and apoptosis (programmed cell death)

Senescence

39) Aging, cellular senescence and cancer. Campisi J. Ann Rev Physiol. 2013; 75: 685-705. doi: 10.1146/annurev-physiol-030212-183653

40) The limited in vitro lifetime of human dipoid cell strains. Hayflick L. Exp Cell Res. 1965; 37: 614-36.

41) The signals and pathways activating cellular senescence. Ben-Porath I, Weinberg RA. Int J Biochem Cell Biol. 2005; 37(5):961-76. epub 2004 Dec 30. doi: 10.1016/j.biocel.2004.10.013

42) Accumulation of short telomeres in human fibroblasts prior to replicative senescence. Martens UM, Chavez EA, Poon SS et al. Exp Cell Res. 2000; 256(1): 291-9. doi:10.1006/excr.2000.4823.

43) Molecular signaling and genetic pathways of senescence: its role in tumorigenesis and aging. Zhang H. J Cell Physiol. 2007;210(3):567-74. doi: 10.1002/jcp.20919

44) Creation of human tumor cells with defined genetic elements. Hahn WC, Counter CM, Lundberg AS et al. Nature. 1999; 400(6743): 464-8. doi:10.1038/22780.

45) Telomeres and telomerase. Chan SRWL, Blackburn EH. Phil. Trans. R. Soc. Lond. 2004; 359: 109-121. doi: 10.1098/rstb.2003.1370

46) Proteinopathy-induced neuronal senescence: a hypothesis for brain failure in Alzheimer's and other neurodegenerative diseases. Golde TE, Miller VM. Alzheimers Res Ther. 2009; 1: 5. doi: 10.1186/alzrt5

Apoptosis

47) Bax monomers form dimer units in the membrane that further self-assemble into multiple oligomeric species. Subburaj Y, Cosentino K, Axmann M et al. Nat Commun. 2015; 6: 8042. doi: 10.1038/ncomms9042

48) DRP-1-mediated mitochondrial fragmentation during EGL-1-induced cell death in C. elegans. Jagasia R, Grote P, Westermann B, Conradt B. Nature. 2005; 433(7027): 754-60. doi: 10.1038/nature03316

Main part 1

Dynamic energy metabolism

49) Mitochondrial dysfunction and oxidative stress in neurodegenerative diseases. Lin MT, Beal MF. Nature. 2006; 443(7113): 787-95. doi: 10.1038/nature05292

50) Oxidative phosphorylation defects and Alzheimer's disease. Shoffner JM. Neurogenetics. 1997; 1:13-9.

The Astrocyte-Neurons-Lactate Shuttle (ANLS) Hypothesis

51) Synaptic energy use and supply. Harris JJ, Jolivet R, Attwell D. Neuron. 2012; 75(5): 762-77. doi:10.1016/j.neuron.2012.08.019.

52) A Cellular Perspective on Brain Energy Metabolism and Functional Imaging. Magistretti PJ, Allaman I. Neuron. 2015; 86(4): 883-901. doi: 10.1016/j.neuron.2015.03.035

53) Glucose and lactate supply to the synapse. Barros LF, Deitmer JW. Brain Res Rev 2010; 63(1-2): 149-59. epub 2009 Oct 30. doi:10.1016/j.brainresrev.2009.10.002.

54) Lactate-supported synaptic function in the rat hippocampal slice preparation. Schurr A, West CA, Rigor BM. Science. 1988; 240(4857): 1326-8.

55) Cell-cell and intracellular lactate shuttles. Brooks G.A. (2009). J Physiol. 2009; 587(23): 5591-5600. doi: 10.1113/jphysiol.2009.178350

Neuroenergetic model

56) An Inverse Warburg effect and the origin of Alzheimer's disease. Demetrius LA, Simon DK. Biogerontology. 2012; 13(6): 583-94. doi:10.1007/s10522-012-9403-6.

57) Energy on demand. Magistretti PJ, Pellerin L, Rothman DL et al. Science. 1999; 283(5401): 496-7.

58) Direct neuronal glucose uptake heralds activity-dependent increases in cerebral metabolism. Lundgaard I, Baoman L, Xie L et al. Nature Com. 2015; 6: 6807. doi: 10.1038/ncomms7807

59) Über den Stoffwechsel der Carcinomzelle. Warburg O. Die Naturwissenschaften. 1924; 12(50): 1131-1137. doi: 10.1007/BF01504608

60) Alzheimer's disease: the amyloid hypothesis and the Inverse Warburg effect. Demetrius LA, Magistretti PJ, Pellerin L. Front Physiol. 2014; 5: 522. doi: 10.3389/fphys.2014.00522

61) Entropy Explains Aging, Genetic Determinism Explains Longevity and Undefined Terminology Explains Misunderstanding Both. Hayflick L. PLoS Genet. 2007; 3(12): e220. doi: 10.1371/journal.pgen.0030220

Side View Warburg Effect, Inverse Warburg effect

62) On the origin of cancer cells. Warburg O. Science. 1956; 123(3191): 309-14.

63) Glutamate uptake into astrocytes stimulates aerobic glycolysis: a mechanism coupling neuronal activity to glucose utilization. Pellerin L, Magistretti PJ. Proc Natl Acad Sci. 1994; 91(22): 10625-10629.

64) Sweet sixteen for ANLS. Pellerin L, Magistretti PJ. J Cereb Blood Flow Metab. 2012; 32(7): 1152-66. epub 2011 Oct 26. doi:10.1038/jcbfm.2011.149.

65) Persistent Mitochondrial Damage by Nitric Oxide and its Derivatives: Neuropathological Implications. Bolaños JP, Heales SJR. Front Neuroenergetics. 2010; 2: 1. Published online 2010. doi: 10.3389/neuro.14.001.2010

Main part 2

Mitochondrial dynamics and developmental aspects.

66) A mitochondrial paradigm of metabolic and degenerative diseases, aging and cancer: a dawn for evolutionary medicine. Wallace DC. Annu Rev Genet. 2005; 39: 359-407. doi: 10.1146/annurev.genet.39.110304.095751

67) Diet impact on mitochondrial bioenergetics and dynamics. Putti R, Raffaella Sica R, Migliaccio V et al. Front Physiol. 2015; 6: 109. doi: 10.3389/fphys.2015.00109

Main part 3

Dynamics of the mtDNA Heteroplasmy and manifestation of diseases / manifestation of diseases.

68) Mitochondrial respiratory-chain diseases. DiMauro S, Schon EA. N Engl J Med. 2003; 348(26):2656-68. doi: 10.1056/NEJMra022567.

69) A mitochondrial bioenergetic etiology of disease. Wallace DC. J Clin Invest. 2013;123(4):1405-1412. doi: 10.1172/JCI61398

70) Mitochondrial threshold effects. Rossignol R, Faustin B, Rocher et al. Biochem J. 2003; 370(Pt 3): 751-762. doi: 10.1042/BJ20021594

71) Mitochondrial DNA mutations and human disease. Tuppen HAL, Blakely EL, Douglass M. et al. Biochimica et Biophysica Acta (BBA) - Bioenergetics. 2010; 1797 (2):113-128. doi: doi.org/10.1016/j.bbabio.2009.09.005.

72) The dynamics of mitochondrial DNA heteroplasmy: implications for human health and disease. Stewart JB, Chinnery PF. Nature Reviews Genetics. 2015; 16: 530-542. doi: 10.1038/nrg3966

Potentially appropriate diagnostic and therapeutic procedures

Pathoetiogenesis of mitochondrial dysfunction / Diagnostic possibilities / Further development of optical information-based biomarkers

73) Review of biomedical optical imaging-a powerful, non-invasive, non-ionizing technology for improving in vivo diagnosis. Balas C. Meas. Sci. Technol. 2009; 20: 104020. doi: 10.1088/0957-0233/20/10/104020

74) Optical sensors for monitoring dynamic changes of intracellular metabolite levels in mammalian cells. Hou BH, Takanaga H, Grossmann G et al. Nature Protocols. 2011; 6:1818-1833. doi: 10.1038/nprot.2011.392

75) Optical sensors for measuring dynamic changes of cytosolic metabolite levels in yeast. Bermejo C, Haerizadeh F, Takanaga H et al. Nature Protocols.2011;6:1806-1817. doi: 10.1038/nprot.2011.391

76) Small is fast: astrocytic glucose and lactate metabolism at cellular resolution. Barros LF, San Martín A, Sotelo-Hitschfeld T et al. Front Cell Neurosci. 2013; 7 :27. doi: 10.3389/fncel.2013.00027

77) In vivo monitoring of cellular energy metabolism using SoNar, a highly responsive sensor for NAD+/NADH redox state. Zhao Y, Aoxue Wang A, Zou Y et al. Nature Protocols. 2016; 11: 1345-1359. doi: 10.1038/nprot.2016.074

78) A Genetically Encoded FRET Lactate Sensor and Its Use To Detect the Warburg Effect in Single Cancer Cells. San Martín A, Ceballo S, Ruminot I, et al. PLoS One. 2013; 8(2): e57712. doi: 10.1371/journal.pone.0057712

Energy metabolism

79) Eine kritische Evaluierung FRET-basierte Biosensoren als Werkzeuge für die quantitative Metabolikanalyse. Moussa R. Schriften des Forschungszentrums Jülich, Reihe Gesundheit / Health, Band / Volume 54. 2012 ISBN 978-3-89336-792-4.

Mitochondrial redox marker

80) In vivo ROS production and use of oxidative stress-derived biomarkers to detect the onset of diseases such as Alzheimer's disease, Parkinson's disease and diabetes. Umeno A, Biju V, Yoshida Y. Free Radic Res. 2017; 51(4): 413-427. doi:10.1080/10715762.2017.1315114.

81) Detection of Reactive Oxygen and Nitrogen Species by Electron Paramagnetic Resonance (EPR) Technique. Suzen S, Hande Gurer-Orhan H; Saso L. Molecules. 2017; 22(1). pii: E181. doi:10.3390/molecules22010181.

82) Glutathione as a Redox Biomarker in mitochondrial disease-Implications for Therapy. Enns GM, Cowan TM. J. Clin. Med. 2017, 6, 50. doi: 10.3390/jcm6050050

Electron acceptors NADH/FAD

83) Intracellular coenzymes as natural biomarkers for metabolic activities and mitochondrial abnormalities. Heikal AA. BioMark Med. 2010; 4(2): 241-263. doi: 10.2217/bmm.10.1.

84) Characterization of Frex as an NADH sensor for in vivo applications in the presence of NAD+ and at various pH values. Wilkening, S., Schmitt, FJ., Horch, M. et al. Photosynth Res.2017. doi:10.1007/s11120-017-0348-0.

Mitochondrial dynamics

85) Abnormal mitochondrial dynamics in the pathogenesis of Alzheimer's disease. Zhu X, Perry G, Smith MA et al. J Alzheimers Dis. 2013; 33 Suppl 1:S253-62. doi: 10.3233/JAD-2012-129005.

86) Mitochondrial Dynamics and Metabolic Regulation. Wai T, Langer T. 2016; 27 (2): 105-117. doi: 10.1016/j.tem.2015.12.001

87) Abnormalities of Mitochondrial Dynamics in Neurodegenerative Diseases. Gao J, Wang L, Liu J et al. Antioxidants. 2017; 6: 25. doi:10.3390/antiox6020025.

88) 3D Time-lapse Imaging and Quantification of Mitochondrial Dynamics. Sison M, Chakrabortty S, Extermann J et al. Scientific Reports. 2017; 7: 43275. doi: 10.1038/srep43275

89) Computational imaging reveals mitochondrial morphology as a biomarker of cancer phenotype and drug response. Giedt RJ, Fumene Feruglio P, Pathania D et al. Sci Rep. 2016; 6: 32985. doi: 10.1038/srep32985

Senescence

90) Are there roles for brain cell senescence in aging and neurodegenerative disorders? Tan FCC, Hutchison ER, Eitan E, et al. Biogerontology. 2014; 6: 643-660. doi: 10.1007/s10522-014-9532-1

91) Senescent Cells. Matjusaitis M, Chin G, Sarnoski EA, et al. Ageing Res Rev. 2016; 29: 1-12. doi: https://doi.org/10.1016/j.arr.2016.05.003

92) Senescence-associated β-galactosidase activity marks the visceral endoderm of mouse embryos but is not indicative of senescence. Huang T, Rivera-Pérez JA. Genesis. 2014;52(4):300-308. published online 2014 doi: 10.1002/dvg.22761

93) Methods to detect biomarkers of cellular senescence: The senescence-associated beta-galactosidase assay. Itahana K, Campisi J, Dimri GP. Methods Mol Biol. 2007; 371: 21-31.

94) Is senescence-associated β-galactosidase a marker of neuronal senescence? Piechota M, Sunderland P, Wysocka A. Oncotarget. 2016; 7(49): 81099-81109. doi:10.18632/oncotarget.12752.

95) Unfolded p53: a potential biomarker for Alzheimer's disease. Lanni C, Uberti D, Racchi M. J. Alzheimer's Dis. 2007; 12: 93-99

Apoptosis/Programmed cell death

96) Programmed Cell Death Mechanisms in Neurological Disease. Bredesen DE. Curr Mol Med.2008; 8(3): 173-186. doi: 10.2174/156652408784221315

97) Targeting programmed cell death in neurodegenerative diseases. Vila M, Przedborski S. Nat Rev Neurosci. 2003; 4 (5), 365-375. doi: 10.1038/nrn1100

98) Cell Death Targets and Potential Modulators in Alzheimers Disease. Castro RE, Santos MMM, Gloria PMC et al. Curr Pharm design. 2010; 16(25): 2851 - 2864. doi: 10.2174/138161210793176563

99) Biomarkers for apoptosis in Alzheimer's disease. Ankarcrona M, Winblad B. Int J Geriatr Psychiatry. 2005; 20(2): 101-200. doi: 10.1002/gps.126

Therapeutic options

100) Comparative Effectiveness and Safety of Cognitive Enhancers for Treating Alzheimer's Disease: systematic review and network metaanalysis. Tricco AC, Ashoor HM, Soobiah C et al. J Am Geriatr Soc. 2017 e-pub- doi: 10.1111/jgs.15069

101) The Transcription Factor Sp3 Cooperates with HDAC2 to Regulate Synaptic Function and Plasticity in Neurons Yamakawa H, Cheng J, Penney J et al. Cell Reports. 2017; 20: 1319-1334. doi: 10.1016/j.celrep.2017.07.044

Multimodal therapy approaches

102) Potential for primary prevention of Alzheimer's disease: an analysis of population-based data. Norton S, Matthews FE, Barnes DE, et al. Lancet Neurology. 2016; 13: 788-794. doi: http://dx.doi.org/10.1016/S1474-4422(14)70136-X

103) A 2-year multidomain intervention of diet, exercise, cognitive training and vascular risk monitoring versus control to prevent cognitive decline in at-risk elderly people (FINGER): a randomised controlled trial. Ngandu T, Lehtisalo J, Solomon A et al. Lancet. 2014; 385: 2255-63. doi: http://dx.doi.org/10.1016/S0140-6736(15)60461-5

104) The Study of Mental and Resistance Training (SMART) study-resistance training and/or cognitive training in mild cognitive impairment: a randomized, double-blind, double-sham controlled trial. Singh F, Gates N, Saigal N et al. J Am Med Dir Assoc. 2014; 15: 873-880. doi: https://doi.org/10.1016/j.jamda.2014.09.010

105) Alzheimer's disease. Scheltens, P, Blennow K, Breteler MMB et al. Lancet. 2016, 388(10043): 505-517. doi: 10.1016/S0140-6736(15)01124-1

106) Nutrition and neurodegeneration: epidemiological evidence and challenges for future research. Gillette-Guyonnet S, Secher M, Vellas B. Br J Clin Pharmacol. 2013; 75(3):738-55. doi: 10.1111/bcp.12058

107) Effect of a Purpose in Life on Risk of Incident Alzheimer Disease and Mild Cognitive Impairment in Community-Dwelling Older Persons. Boyle, PA; Buchman AS, MD; Lisa L. Barnes LL et al. Arch Gen Psychiatry. 2010; 67(3): 304-310. doi: 10.1001/archgenpsychiatry.2011.1487

108) Mitohormesis: Promoting Health and Lifespan by Increased Levels of Reactive Oxygen Species (ROS). Ristow M, Schmeisser K. Dose Response. 2014; 12(2): 288-341. doi: 10.2203/dose-response.13-035.Ristow

109) Mitochondrial Dysfunction in Alzheimer's Disease and the Rationale for Bioenergetics Based Therapies. Isaac G. Onyango IG, Dennis J et al. Aging Dis. 2016 Mar; 7(2): 201-214. doi: 10.14336/AD.2015.1007

Metabolic interventions

110) Lactate-mediated glia-neuronal signaling in the mammalian brain. Tang F, Lane S, Korsak A, et al. Nat Commun. 2014; 5: 3284. doi: 10.1038/ncomms4284

111) The role of Lactate-mediated metabolic coupling between Astrocytes and Neurons in long-term memory formation. Front Integr Neurosci. 2016; 10: Article 10. Steinman MQ, Gao V, Alberini CM. doi: 10.3389/fnint.2016.00010

112) Medium-chain fatty acids inhibit mitochondrial metabolism in astrocytes promoting astrocyte-neuron lactate and ketone body shuttle systems. Thevenet J, Marchi U, Santo Domingo J et al. FASEB J. 2016; 5: 1913-26. doi: 10.1096/fj.201500182

Mitochondrial dynamics

113) Mitochondrial fusion and fission proteins: novel therapeutic targets for combating cardiovascular disease. Hall AR, Burke N, Dongworth RK et al. Br J Pharmacol. 2014; 171 (8):1890-906. doi: 10.1111/bph.12516
Homo and heteroplasmy, CrisprCas9 technology and gene replacement therapy

114) CRISPR/Cas9 and mitochondrial gene replacement therapy: promising techniques and ethical considerations. Fogleman S, Santana C, Bishop C et al. Am J Stem Cells. 2016; 5(2): 39-52.

115) Live birth derived from oocyte spindle transfer to prevent mitochondrial disease Zhang J, Hui L, Shiyu L et al. Reproductive Biomedicine online:2017;34(4):361-368. doi: 10.1016/j.rbmo.2017.01.013

New view on the Neurodegeneration of the sporadic form of Alzheimer's disease

Evolutive environmental interactions / Inverse Warburg effect / consequences of mtDNA-mutations: Senescence and programmed cell death / Consequences of a disturbed protein quality control

116) The large Hsp70 Grp170 binds to unfolded protein substrates in vivo with a regulation distinct from conventional Hsp70s. Behnke J, Hendershot LM. J Biol Chem. 2014; 289(5): 2899-907. epub 2013 Dec 10. doi: 10.1074/jbc.M113.507491

117) Intracellular amyloid-beta in Alzheimer's disease. LaFerla FM, Green KN, Oddo S. Nat Rev Neurosci. 2007; 8(7): 499-509. doi: 10.1038/nrn2168

118) The Genetics of Alzheimer Disease Tanzi RE. Cold Spring Harb Perspect Med. 2012; 2(10): a006296. doi: 10.1101/cshperspect.a006296

119) Amyloid-β peptide induces mitochondrial dysfunction by inhibition of preprotein maturation. Mossmann D, Vögtle FN, Taskin AA et al. Cell Metab. 2014; 20(4): 662-9. doi: 10.1016/j.cmet.2014.07.024

Energetic-genetic correlation

Brain plasticity

120) Healthy aging and dementia: Findings from the Nun Study. Snowdon D. Ann Intern Med. 2003; 139: 450-454.

121) The Nun Study Iacono D, Markesbery WR, Gross M et al: Neurology. 2009;73(9): 665-673. doi: 10.1212/WNL.0b013e3181b01077

122) Alzheimer's disease is a synaptic failure. Selkoe DJ. Science. 2002; 298(5594): 789-91. doi:10.1126/science.1074069.

123) Mitochondrial Dysfunction and Synaptic Transmission Failure in Alzheimer's disease. Guo L, Tian J, Du H. J. Alzheimers Dis. 2017; 57(4): 1071-1086. doi: 10.3233/JAD-160702

Healthy and pathological aging

124) Family member deaths across adulthood predict Alzheimer's Disease risk. The Cache County Study. Norton MC, Elizabeth Fauth E, Clark CJ et al. Int J Geriatr Psychiatry. 2016; 31(3): 256-263. doi: 10.1002/gps.4319

125) Post-stroke dementia - a comprehensive review. Mijajlović MD, Pavlović A, Brainin Met al. BMC Med. 2017; 15:11. doi: 10.1186/s12916-017-0779-7

126) Heart failure and Alzheimer's disease. Cermakova P, Eriksdotter M, Lu LH et al. J Intern Med 2015; 277(4): 406-425. doi: 10.1111/joim.12287

127) Head Injury as a Risk Factor for Dementia and Alzheimer's Disease: A Systematic Review and Meta-Analysis of 32 Observational Studies. Li Ya, Li Yo, Li X et al. PLoS One. 2017; 12(1): e0169650. doi: 10.1371/journal.pone.0169650

128) The significance of environmental factors in the etiology of Alzheimer's disease. Grant WB, Campbell A, Itzhaki RF et al. J Alzheimers Dis. 2002; 4(3): 179-89.

129) Rate of death among family members predicts risk of Alzheimer's disease and other dementias: The Cache County study. Norton M, Roxane Pfister R, Mineau G et al. Alzheimer's & Dementia. 2011; 7(4)Suppl: 599

130) Links between life events, traumatism and dementia; an open study including 565 patients with dementia. Charles E, Bouby-Serieys V, Thomas P et al. Encephale. 2006; 32(5 Pt 1): 746-52.

Result and conclusions
Another view on the origin of the sporadic form of Alzheimer's disease / Quantum biological background / From biological quantum physics to Quantum Biology

131) Quantisierung als Eigenwertproblem (Erste Mitteilung). Schrödinger E. Annalen der Physik.1926;79(4):361-376.

Quantisierung als Eigenwertproblem (Zweite Mitteilung). Schrödinger E. Annalen der Physik,1926;79(4):489-527.

Quantisierung als Eigenwertproblem (Dritte Mitteilung). Perturbation theory, with application to the Stark effect of Balmer lines. Schrödinger E. Annalen der Physik.1926;80(4):437-490.

Quantisierung als Eigenwertproblem (Vierte Mitteilung). Schrödinger E. Annalen der Physik.1926;81(4):109-139.

132) Generelle Morphologie der Organismen. Allgemeine Grundzüge der Organismen. Allgemeine Grunzüge der organischen Formen - Wissenschft, mechanisch begründet durch die von Charles Darwin reformierte Descendenz-Theorie. Haeckel E. Georg Reimer, Berlin 1866

133) The Descent of Man (1879). Darwin C. Penguin Books 2004. ISBN-13 978-0-140-43631-0

134) Versuche über Pflanzenhybride. Mendel JG. In: Verhandlungen des Naturforschenden Vereines in Brünn. Vol. IV. 1866: 3-47.

135) Über den anschaulichen Inhalt der quantentheoretischen Kinematik und Mechanik. Heisenberg W. Zeitschrift für Physik. 1927; 3 (43): 172-198. doi:10.1007/BF01397280.

136) Die fraktale Geometrie der Natur. Mandelbrot B. Birkhäuser Basel; Springer Basel AG 1987. ISBN 978-3-0348-5028-5.

137) Making Sense of Bell's Theorem and Quantum Nonlocality. Boughn S. Princeton University, Princeton NJ 08544. Haverford College, Haverford PA 19041 Found Phys. 2017; 47: 640. 2017 arXiv:1703.11003 doi: 10.1007/s10701-017-0083-6

138) Quantenbiologie. Einführung in einen neuen Wissenszweig. Dessauer F. Springer-Verlag Berlin, Göttingen, Heidelberg. 1954

139) Die Physik und das Geheimnis des organischen Lebens. Jordan P. Friedrich Vieweg und Sohn Braunschweig. 1941

140) Die Quantenmechanik und die Grundprobleme der Biologie und Psychologie. Jordan P. Natural Sciences 1932; 20 (45): 815-821.
doi: 10.1007/BF01494844

141) Was ist Leben? Schrödinger E. R. Piper GmbH & Co. KG Munich 1987. ISBN 3-492-11134-3

142) Vibrations, Quanta and Biology. Huelga SF, Plenio MB. Contemp. Phys. 2013; 54: 181 - 207. doi: 10.1080/00405000.2013.829687

Physical reality and Realness
From statistical-physical to elementary information: Bits and Qubits

143) Dialog mit der Natur. Prigogine I. R Piper Verlag Munich. 1990. ISBN 3-492-11181-5

144) Physik der Selbstorganisation und Evolution. Ebeling W, Feistel R. Akademie Verlag Berlin. 1982: 83 ff.

145) A Mathematical Theory of Information. Shannon CE: In: Bell System Technical Journal. Short Hills N.J. 27.1948: 379 - 423, 623 - 656. 1948 ISSN 0005-8580.

Relationship between quantum information and measurement process

146) Die Quantentheorie der einfachen Alternative (Komplementarität und Logik II). Weizsäcker CFv. Z. Naturforschg. 1958; 13 a: 705-721.

147) Die Einheit der Natur. Weizsäcker CFv. Hanser Verlag Munich 1981, ISBN 3-446-12743-7.

148) Quantum Field Theory of Binary Alternatives. Görnitz T, Graudenz D, Weizsäcker CFv. Intern. J. Theoret. Phys. 1992; 31: 1929-1959.

149) Deriving General Relativity from Considerations on Quantum Information. Görnitz T. Adv. Sci. Lett. 2011; 4: 577-585. doi: 10.1166/asl.2011.1243

Interactions in the living via bit and qubit

150) Experimental Quantum Teleportation. Bouwmeester D, Pan JW, Mattle K et al. Nature. 1997; 390: 575-579. doi: 10.1038/37539

151) Was ist Krankheit? Quanteneffekte in der Medizin. Wrobel N, Sedlacek KD. BoD Books on Demand, Norderstedt. 2015: 163ff. ISBN 978-3-7347-9263-2

Novel measurement methods as biophysical Biomarkers

152) Was ist Krankheit? Quanteneffekte in der Medizin. Wrobel N, Sedlacek KD. Bod Books on Demand, Norderstedt. 2015: 214ff. ISBN 978-3-7347-9263-2

Possibilities of an entropy- or information-based diagnostics / possibilities of quantum physics-based diagnostics / fluorescence resonance energy transfer

153) Zwischenmolekulare Energiewanderung und Fluoreszenz. Förster, T. Ann. Phys.(1948) 437: 55-75. doi:10.1002/andp.19484370105.

Electron transport by Porphyrins

154) The quantum tunneling effect leads electron transport in porphyrins. Spanish National Research Council (CSIC). EurekAlert, Public Release. 2011 eurekalert.org/pub_releases/2011-09/ccsd-tqt090111.php

155) Über quantenmechanische Energieübertragungen zwischen atomaren Systemen. Kallmann H, London F. Z. Phys. Chem. 1928; B. 2: 207-243.

Principle detection of quantum effects in the hemoglobin
Are diagnostically and therapeutically integrated procedures possible in principle?

156) Interaction-Free Measurement. Kwiat P, Weinfurter H, Herzog T et al. Phys. Rev. Lett. 1995; 74: 4763. doi: 10.1103/PhysRevLett.74.4763

157) Interaction-free measurement study as a quantum channel discrimination problem. Zhou Y, Yung M-H. 2017 arXiv:1703.03976.

158) A new theory of the origin of cancer: quantum coherentanglement, centrioles, mitosis and differentiation. Hameroff SR. Biosystems. 2004; 77(1-3): 119-36.

159) DNA as classical and quantum information system: implication to gene expression in normal and cancer cells. Koruga D. Arch Oncol 2005;13(3-4):115-20. doi: 10.2298/AOO0503115K

160) Quantum information processing at the cellular level. Euclidean approach. Ogryzko V. Institute Gustave Roussy, Villejuif, France. 2009 arxiv.org/abs/0906.4279

How might human life function according to quantum biological principles?

Pure and everyday coincidence / Evolutive Awareness

161) The origin of mutants. Cairns, J; Overbaugh J; Miller S. Nature. 1988; 335: 142-45. doi: 10.1038/335142a0

162) Quantum Zeno effect in a double-well potential: A model of a physical measurement. Altenmüller TP, Schenzle A. Phys. Rev. 1994; 3(49): 2016-2027 doi: 10.1103/PhysRevA.49.2016

Integrity of the biological space-time construction
Life between health and disease

163) Was ist Krankheit? Quanteneffekte in der Medizin. Wrobel N, Sedlacek KD. Bod Books on Demand, Norderstedt. 2015: 220ff. ISBN 978-3-7347-9263-2

The mitochondrial energy aspect from a quantum biological perspective:

The quantum mitochondrion

164) Mitochondrial Oscillations in Physiology and Pathophysiology. Aon MA, Cortassa S, O'Rourke B. Adv Exp Med Biol. 2008; 641: 98-117. doi: 10.1007/978-0-387-09794-7

165) Quantum electron tunneling in respiratory complex I. Hayashi T, Stuchebrukhov AA. J. Phys Chem. B. 2011;115:5354-5364. doi: 10.1021/jp109410j

166) Electron tunneling chains of mitochondria. Moser CC, Farid TA, Chobot SE et al. Biochim. Biophys. Acta. 2006;1757:1096-1109. doi: 10.1016/j.bbabio.2006.04.015

Electron transport chain

167) MoleculaMolekularbiologie der Zelle. Alberts B, Johnson A, Lewis J et al. New York: John Wiley & Sons. 2011: 935ff. ISBN: 978-3-527-32384-5

Enzymes

168) Towards a new biochemistry? Szent-Gyorgyi A. Science. 1941;93: 609-611. doi: 10.1126/science.93.2426.609

169) Studies of photosynthesis using a pulsed laser. Temperature dependence of cytochrome oxidation rate in chromatium. Evidence for tunneling. DeVault D, Chance B. Biophys. J. 1966; 6 :825-847. doi: 10.1016/S0006-3495(66)86698-5

170) Kinetic isotope effects as a probe of hydrogen transfers to and from common enzymatic cofactors. Roston D., Islam Z., Kohen A. Arch. Biochem. Biophys. 2014; 544: 96-104. doi: 10.1016/j.abb.2013.10.010

171) Enzyme dynamics and hydrogen tunnelling in a thermophilic alcohol dehydrogenase. Kohen A, Cannio R, Bartolucci S, Klinman JP. Nature. 1999; 399: 496-499. doi: 10.1038/ 20981

172) Vibronic origin of long-lived coherence in an artificial molecular light harvester. Lim J, Paleček D, Caycedo-Soler F et al. Nature Com. 2015; 6: Article number: 7755. doi :10.1038/ncomms8755.

Mitochondrial dynamics (fusion and fission)

173) Mitochondrial filaments and clusters as intracellular power-transmitting cables. Skulachev VP. Trends Biochem. Sci. 2001;26:23-29. doi: 10.1016/S0968-0004(00)01735-7

174) Electric field-induced fusion of mitochondria. Reynaud JA, Labbe H, Lequoc K et al. FEBS Lett. 1989;247:106-112. doi: 10.1016/0014-5793(89)81250-5

175) Frohlich systems in cellular physiology. Srobar F. Prague. Med. rep. 2012;113:95-104. doi: 10.14712/23362936.2015.25

176) Effect of calcium on electrical energy transfer by microtubules. Priel A, Ramos AJ, Tuszynski JA et al. J. Biol. Phys. 2008;34:475-485. doi: 10.1007/s10867-008-9106-z

DNA mutation

177) Proton tunneling in DNA and its biological implications. Löwdin PO. Rev. Mod. Phys. 1963; 35, 724-732. doi: 10.1103/RevModPhys.35.724

178) Roles of evolution, quantum mechanics and point mutations in origins of cancer. Cooper WG. Cancer Biochem Biophys. 1993; 13(3): 147-70.

179) Quantum Effects and Genetic Code: Dynamics and Information Transfer in DNA Replication. S. Mayburov S, Nicolini C, Sivozhelezov V. Lebedev Inst. of Physics Leninski, Moscow, Russia, 117924. 2006 arxiv.org/ftp/q-bio/papers/0611/0611009.pdf.

180) Correlated quantum transport of density wave electrons. Miller JH, Wijesinghe AI, Tang Z et al. Phys Rev Lett. 2012;108(3):036404. Epub 2012. doi: 10.1103/PhysRevLett.108.036404

181) Quantum entanglement between the electron clouds of nucleic acids in DNA. Rieper E anders J, Vedral V. Center for Quantum Technologies, National University of Singapore, Republic of Singapore. 2011 arxiv.org/abs/1006.4053

182) Entanglement at the quantum phase transition in a harmonic lattice. Rieper E anders J, Vedral V. New J. Phys. 2010; 12: Articel 025017. doi: 10.1103/PhysRevD.86.125011

183) Photolyase/cryptochrome blue-light photoreceptors use photon energy to repair DNA and reset the circadian clock. Thompson CL, Sancar A. Oncogene. 2002; 21, 9043-9056. doi: 10.1038/sj.onc.1205958

184) Quantum entanglement in photosynthetic light-harvesting complexes. Sarovar M, Ishizaki A, Fleming GR et al. Nature Physics. 2010; 6: 462-467. doi: 10.1038/nphys1652

Reactive oxygen species (ROS)

185) The Quantum Biology of Reactive Oxygen Species Partitioning Impacts Cellular Bioenergetics. Usselman RJ, Chavarriaga C, Castello PR et al. Scientific Reports 2016; 6: 38543. doi: 10.1038/srep38543

Protein folding

186) Electron tunneling through proteins. Gray, HB, Winkler JR. Q Rev Biophys. 2003; 36(3):3 41-72.

Do aware processes check protein quality control?

187) Atomic-Level Characterization of the Structural Dynamics of Proteins. Shaw DE, Maragakis P, Lindorff-Larsen K. Science. 2010. 330 (6002): 341-346. doi: 10.1126/science.1187409

The importance of pure chance

188) Variation in cancer risk among tissues can be explained by the number of stem cell divisions. Tomasetti C, Vogelstein B. Science. 2015; 347(6217): 78-81. doi: 10.1126/science.1260825

189) Commentary: The age distribution of cancer and a multistage theory of carcinogenesis. Doll R. Int J Epidemiol. 2004;33(6):1183-4. epub 2004 Nov 2. doi: 10.1093/ije/dyh359

Summary and outlook

190) Quantum Tunneling to the Origin and Evolution of Life. Trixler F. Curr Org Chem. 2013; 17(16): 1758-1770. doi: 10.2174/13852728113179990083

191) A quantum mechanical model of adaptive mutation. McFadden J, Al-Khalili J. Biosystems. 1999; 50(3): 203-11.

9 Index